LEARNING
SOLUTION-FOCUSED
THERAPY
An Illustrated Guide

LEARNING
SOLUTION-FOCUSED
THERAPY
An Illustrated Guide

By

Anne Bodmer Lutz, B.S.N., M.D.

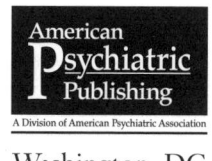

American **P**sychiatric Publishing

A Division of American Psychiatric Association

Washington, DC
London, England

Copyright © 2014 American Psychiatric Association
ALL RIGHTS RESERVED

Manufactured in the United States of America on acid-free paper
17   16   15   14   13   5   4   3   2   1
First Edition
Typeset in Janson text LT Std and Frutiger LT Std.

American Psychiatric Publishing
A Division of American Psychiatric Association
1000 Wilson Boulevard
Arlington, VA 22209-3901
www.appi.org

Library of Congress Cataloging-in-Publication Data
Lutz, Anne Bodmer, 1963- author.
  Learning solution-focused therapy : an illustrated guide / by Anne Bodmer Lutz. -- First edition.
      p. ; cm.
  Includes bibliographical references and index.
  ISBN 978-1-58562-452-2 (pbk. : alk. paper)
  I. Title.
  [DNLM: 1. Psychotherapy, Brief--methods. 2. Professional-Patient Relations. WM 420.5.P5]
  RC480.5
  616.89′14--dc23
                                                                          2013024819

British Library Cataloguing in Publication Data
A CIP record is available from the British Library.

Contents

Video Illustrations: www.appi.org/Lutz

About the Author

Anne Bodmer Lutz, M.D., is the Director of Training of the Institute for Solution-Focused Therapy. She is a board certified adult and child and adolescent psychiatrist and was a nurse prior to becoming a physician. She was trained by the founders of solution-focused therapy, Insoo Kim Berg and Steve De Shazer, and has provided training seminars with Insoo Kim Berg and Yvonne Dolan.

Dr. Lutz is an assistant professor of psychiatry at the University of Massachusetts, Worcester. She is also the medical director of a residential treatment center for adolescent girls suffering from addiction and co-occurring disorders that integrates solution-focused approaches within its treatment setting. She provides direct clinical supervision, teaching, and training to psychiatric residents and psychology interns, as well as workshops for community-based treatment organizations. She also has a private practice in which she sees children and families, providing solution-focused psychiatric treatment.

Dr. Lutz has both worked and provided solution-focused trainings in a wide variety of treatment settings integrating solution-focused approaches, including community mental health centers, schools, youth violence prevention initiatives, adolescent addiction programs, child and family treatment settings, and psychopharmacotherapy. She lives in Massachusetts with her husband and two sons.

Preface

Solution-focused brief therapy has been steadily growing in influence since the 1970s. It is an evidence-based practice that focuses on creating conversations that build solutions, in contrast to solving problems. This is a book about how to practice solution-focused therapy. My goal in writing this book is to provide an easy-to-use guide to learning the essentials of solution-focused therapy that will assist the reader in becoming competent in this treatment method. The book is written in an informal, conversational style. Chapter 1 begins by providing an overview of the assumptions and tenets used in solution-focused therapy as well as a case review and case illustration. Chapters 2–8 are organized around how an interview is conducted. The last chapters focus on how to apply this model in psychopharmacotherapy, addiction, supervision, and consultation.

The first three chapters introduce skills used when commencing an interview, including beginning with strengths and resources, developing a yes-set, and maintaining meticulous use of language. Chapters 5, 6, and 7 present skills used when negotiating goals, amplifying ambivalence, and dealing with crisis. Chapter 8 presents solution-focused assessment techniques. These chapters combine didactic readings, solution-focused questions, case illustrations, learning exercises, and video illustrations. The case illustrations are filled with detailed explanations in order to help the reader learn how to practice this model of treatment. To help the reader, these explanations are in italics.

Chapters 9 and 10 present ways to apply solution-focused techniques when prescribing medications and when treating patients suffering from addiction. Chapters 11 and 12 describe how to use solution-focused techniques when providing supervision and consultation. In these chapters and throughout the book, learning exercises, videos, and case illustrations are provided.

The videos that accompany the book illustrate key features of solution-focused therapy. The video illustrations are brief vignettes that feature the work of volunteer clinicians who agreed to demonstrate commonly used solution-focused techniques. All case and video illustrations are based on amalgams and experience of treating people with similar problems. The genders, background information, and other data have been changed. The video and case illustrations are described more fully in the Video Guide beginning on page xiii.

I would like to explain a few semantic issues and linguistic conventions used in this book. In dialog with patients, there are times when I use the terms *suffering from* and *struggling with*. My goal in using these phrases is not to represent patients as victims or as objects of pity, but rather to convey empathy, and to communicate that the patient's identity exists apart from and beyond symptomatology. I also choose to use this language so that I talk "about" patients in the same manner that I talk "to" them, maintaining the eminently respectful stance of this treatment approach. In discussing techniques, I choose to use the words *diagnosing strengths* rather than *identifying, discovering,* or *determining* strengths. I think the word usage "diagnosing strengths" more accurately implies that this is a very different way of evaluating and "diagnosing" patients, and communicates the differences of this treatment approach more effectively.

Thank you for choosing to read this book. I hope it will be useful for you, and that you and your patients will benefit from this treatment approach. I hope that the book can be useful to a wide audience as a way to teach solution-focused therapy to undergraduates, graduate students, medical students, and residents and to assist those working in medical practice settings, mental health agencies, and other social service agencies.

Anne Bodmer Lutz, B.S.N., M.D.

Acknowledgments

I am indebted to many teachers and colleagues for their ideas that are incorporated in *Learning Solution-Focused Therapy*, especially the late Steve de Shazer and the late Insoo Kim Berg, of the Brief Family Therapy Center in Milwaukee, Wisconsin, whose life and work profoundly changed my life. I thank Yvonne Dolan of the Institute for Solution-Focused Therapy, whose support, encouragement, words of wisdom were invaluable as she brainstormed, listened, and provided immeasurable help every step of the way. I am blessed to have such an amazing mentor and friend. I thank Terry Trepper of the Institute for Solution-Focused Therapy, whose intelligence, guidance, and vision were invaluable. I thank Dr. Ruth Westheimer, M.D., for her ongoing support and encouragement, and for her belief in my ability to succeed when I didn't think I could. Her support has been inestimable. I thank all the many people who have written extensively about and taught me how to practice solution-focused therapy. I thank my sister, Sylvia Bodmer True, for her encouragement all along the way. My thanks also go to my patients, friends, students, colleagues, and workshop participants whose questions and struggles are the inspiration for much of what has been written. I thank all my colleagues and friends whose names appear in the Video Guide section for volunteering to be actors in the videos. You were all so amazing, talented, and generous!

Finally, I thank my husband, John, and my two children, Ethan and Brandon. They have been incredibly supportive and patient during all the time it took to write this book. My gratitude cannot be summarized in a few sentences. I am so blessed to have you in my life. I cannot imagine a more supportive and loving family. I look forward to our journey together.

Video Guide

In addition to the case illustrations in the chapters, a collection of video vignettes illustrates key skills. These brief videos feature the work of volunteer clinicians who agreed to demonstrate commonly used solution-focused techniques.

▶ **Video Illustration:** Video cues provided in the text identify the vignettes by title and run time.

The videos can be viewed online by navigating to www.appi.org/Lutz and using the embedded video player. The videos are optimized for most current operating systems, including mobile operating systems iOS 5.1 and Android 4.1 and higher.

Video Vignettes

Chapter 2. Beginning With Strengths and Resources

- Beginning with problem-free talk (2:16)
- Identifying VIPs (1:08)
- Identifying and amplifying positive differences (2:16)

Chapter 3. The Yes-Set

- Building the content yes-set (1:38)
- Building the emotional yes-set (1:04)

Chapter 4. Language Skills in Solution-Focused Therapy

- Attention to language (1:10)
- Bridging statements (1:37)

Video Credits

Deepest thanks and appreciation to the clinicians and others who contributed to the videos as actors and as standby volunteers:

Melanie Amir, M.S., OTR/L, Program Director, Highland Grace House, Worcester, Massachusetts

Jamie Carroll, Psy.D., Clinical psychology predoctoral intern

Ebony Coney, Psy.D., Clinical psychology predoctoral intern

Susan Gutwillig, Residential counselor, Highland Grace House

Andrea Henry, Residential counselor, Highland Grace House

Cynthia Keeley, Residential counselor, Highland Grace House

Ethan Lutz

John Lutz, Psy.D., Clinical psychologist, Lutz Child and Family Associates

Abby Mudd, Residential counselor, Highland Grace House

Erica O'Mahoney

Stephanie Roy

Justin Snook

Rachel Stein, D.O., Child psychiatry fellow, University of Massachusetts

Crystal Torres, Residential counselor, Highland Grace House

Sylvia Bodmer True

Kerry Wilkins, M.D., Child psychiatry fellow, University of Massachusetts

James Yon, M.D., Child psychiatry fellow, University of Massachusetts

CHAPTER 1

Introduction to Solution-Focused Therapy

Physicians, and psychiatrists in particular, are in a unique and privileged position to engage patients in conversations that have incredible power to heal. Solution-focused therapy is a competency-based model that minimizes emphasis on past problems and failings and instead focuses on the patient's strengths and prior successes. This treatment approach is in accord with the positive psychology movement that emphasizes well-being and optimal functioning instead of pathology and etiology. Positive psychology is the scientific study of positive experiences, positive individual traits, and the institutions that facilitate their development; it is a discipline concerned with well-being and optimal functioning. Positive psychology differs from the pathology- and etiology-focused medical model in that it focuses instead on resources and strengths. "It's a build what's strong approach supplementing a fix what's wrong approach" (Lee Duckworth et al. 2005, p. 631). Solution-focused therapy focuses on the specifics of how to put this into practice.

A solution-focused approach provides an additive dimension to the problem-focused techniques taught within medicine, and psychiatry in particular, in which there is an expectation that change can occur only through the understanding and exploration of problems. Solution-focused therapy is a competency-based model that directs patients toward their preferred future and strengths instead of their past problems and failings (De Jong and Berg 1998): "Rather than looking for what is wrong and how to fix it, we tend to look for what is right and how to use it" (Berg and Miller 1992, p. 3). This mode of therapy often results in briefer lengths of treatment, and as such it is an essential skill for a child psychiatrist, whose services are in extremely short supply and high demand.

As physicians and psychiatrists are challenged to work with fewer resources while managing and treating increasingly complex and "multiproblem" families, delving into the details of strengths and resources is invaluable. The solution-focused approach was developed, in fact, at a family center, through the work of Steve de Shazer, the late Insoo Kim Berg, and their colleagues at the Brief Family Therapy Center in Milwaukee, Wisconsin (Berg and Miller 1992; De Jong and Berg 1998).

Because so much has been written about problem-focused assessments, the emphasis in this book is on solution-focused assessments. This skill set will provide an additive dimension to the problem-focused assessments predominantly taught in the field of medicine, and particularly in psychiatry. This book will teach the basic tenets of solution-focused therapy, the core skills and techniques required in practicing this model of treatment, and, most critically, the "how-tos" of becoming a solution-focused clinician.

How do people solve problems and create change in their lives? Various answers often emerge when this question is posed. Responses include identifying what the problem is, uncovering the root cause, talking about it, and developing an action plan. However, for a problem to get solved, ultimately something must be done, and in general done differently. Doing more of the same perpetuates the problem, and this is the very reason patients seek help.

de Shazer was a pioneer in the idea that there is not a necessary connection between problem and solution (de Shazer and Berg 1997). He had what seems to many the shocking notion that "solutions need not be directly related to the problems they are meant to solve" (de Shazer 1988). Problems do not happen all the time, and problem patterns are never rigidly fixed through time and across different situations. The fact that a person is aware there is a problem suggests he or she is making a comparison to another time or situation when the problem did not exist. People are people! People generally do things for good reasons, and usually because in some way their behaviors are helpful for them. When patients seek help, things they are doing are no longer working or helpful for them. Something has changed. Either the problem has worsened or they themselves or people around them are more troubled by the problem. When problem focused, the therapist talks with the patient about problems and problem solving. When solution focused, the therapist talks about changes that make a difference and about solutions, rather than about difficulties, complaints, and problems (de Shazer 1985).

In order for problems to be considered solved, one of two things must happen: either the problem no longer occurs or it is no longer viewed as a problem. The techniques practiced using solution-focused therapy help to guide patients toward creating greater awareness of what they want to be different in their lives, uncovering what they are doing differently when things are working in their lives and what they can do differently to accomplish their desired goals. This challenges the clinician to learn skills that will help a patient recognize and identify times when the problem is not occurring and how these successes are being accomplished. These successful times are called positive differences or exceptions, and identifying them requires meticulous listening skills on the part of the physician (De Jong and Berg 1998). These moments are not to be forgotten, ignored, or considered flukes. They are critical periods in which a patient is already having some success, even though often as yet unaware of it. Encouraging patients to do more of these behaviors is pivotal in helping them attain their goals. This is the quintessential principle of the solution-focused therapy model of treatment. If it works, do more of it. If it isn't working, do something different!

The developers of solution-focused therapy were most interested in what works in therapy and how to do therapy. The solution-focused therapy approach was developed inductively based on 30 years of sessions with patients. Together with their colleagues, Insoo Kim Berg and Steve de Shazer watched and videotaped hundreds of sessions with patients, closely observing what works, what questions are helpful, and what techniques and skills promote positive change in patients (de Shazer 1988; de Shazer et al. 1986). This model has been influenced by the work of many others, including Milton Erickson, John Weakland, Paul Watzlawick, Richard Fisch, and Carl Rogers (de Shazer 1988; de Shazer et al. 1986; Erickson 2009a, 2009b; Rogers 1986; Watzlawick et al. 1990). It has been used successfully with a variety of patient populations, including groups, couples, and children, in rehabilitation centers, child protection agencies, community mental health settings, schools, inpatient settings, domestic violence and substance abuse centers, trauma and sexual abuse treatment settings, medical settings, and private practice (Berg 1994; Berg and Miller 1992; Dolan 1991; Franklin et al. 2008; Hoyt and Berg 1998; Iveson et al. 2012; Kelly and Bluestone-Miller 2009; Metcalf 1998; Nelson 2011; Pichot and Smock 2009; Roeden et al. 2009; Selekman 1997, 2008; Simon 2010; Stith et al. 2011; Tews-Kozlowski 2012; Ziegler and Hiller 2007). Many others continue to develop this model of treatment (Franklin et al. 2008; Furman and Ahola 1992; Holyoake and Golding 2012; Iveson et al. 2012; Kim et al. 2010; Sell 2011; Sharry et al. 2012; Trepper et al. 2006).

Solution-focused therapy provides practical techniques that strengthen the therapeutic alliance while detecting and magnifying patients' strengths, resources, and successes. Lambert concluded that as much as 40% of the improvement in psychotherapy is attributable to patient variables and extratherapeutic influences, 30% of effective therapy is due to the therapeutic relationship, 15% to expectancy (placebo effects), and 15% to techniques (Lambert 2001, 2005; Lambert and Barley 2001). Attention to these factors is crucial for effective therapy. Lambert also found that patients who do better in psychotherapy and maintain treatment gains believe that the changes made in therapy were primarily a result of their own efforts (Lambert 2005). Bernes (2005) suggests that basic capacities of human relating—warmth, affirmation, and a minimum of attack and blame—may be at the center of effective psychotherapeutic intervention. The skills developed when practicing solution-focused therapy facilitate these essential capacities: identifying and amplifying positive patient factors, enhancing the therapeutic alliance, promoting self-efficacy, affirming the patient, and attending to extratherapeutic factors (the patient's social context).

Solution-focused therapy can be conceptualized as a meta-model, and when done well it can be integrated with other treatment approaches that all work toward promoting effective treatment and helping patients attain their goals. As noted, solution-focused therapy can be summarized as paying attention to what works and doing more of it, and when things are not working, doing something different (de Shazer 1985). This sounds simple, and indeed in concept it is; however, simple does not mean easy, and applying this approach well can be likened to learning a new language; it requires practice, skill, and persistence.

Solution-focused therapy has considerable empirical support and is firmly grounded in research evidence (Franklin 2012). The following are the basic tenets that inform solution-focused therapy (Franklin 2012):

1. It is based on solution building rather than problem solving.
2. The therapeutic focus is on the patient's desired future rather than on past problems or current conflicts.
3. Patients are encouraged to increase the frequency of current useful behaviors.
4. No problem happens all the time. There are exceptions; that is, there are times when the problem could have happened but didn't. These exceptions can be used by the patient and therapist to co-construct solutions.
5. Therapists help patients find alternatives to current undesired patterns of behavior, cognition, and interaction that are within the patient's repertoire or can be constructed by therapist and patient.
6. Differing from skill building and behavior interventions, the model assumes that solution behaviors already exist for patients and can be discovered by conversation between the therapist and patient.

7. Small increments of change lead to large increments of change.
8. Patients' solutions are not necessarily directly related to any problem identified by either the patient or the therapist.
9. The conversational skills required of the therapist to invite the patient to build solutions are different from those needed to diagnose and treat the patient's problems.

As the name suggests, solution-focused therapy is defined by its emphasis on solutions, and the clinician gives less attention to defining or understanding presenting problems. This is not to minimize or deny the problems—and in fact practicing solution-focused techniques does uncover the problems and symptoms—but the narrative created with the patient uncovers and enhances his or her competencies, strengths, and successes. In traditional problem-focused therapy, the clinician serves as expert, and a thorough understanding of the problem and symptoms is necessary before treatment begins. Traditional problem-focused therapy involves evaluating and diagnosing the problem, using information known about the diagnosed problem, evaluating strengths and resources, and then developing and implementing a treatment plan. Identifying the problem and its root cause are at the core of problem solving. In contrast, solution building takes a radically different approach to evaluating and working with patients. In this model, the clinician works toward helping patients create detailed descriptions of their goals and best hopes for their preferred future, uncovering critical resources and strengths with which they are already having success but of which they not yet aware (Franklin 2012).

This book welcomes you to the challenging and rewarding process of becoming a solution-focused clinician. The reader will learn how to become an expert at searching for clues that reveal hidden strengths and potential resources, rather than deeper problems and hidden pathology, and how to co-create and sustain conversations that amplify patient strengths and resources while helping patients attain their goals. Good diagnosticians know how to look differently at the facts. They know how to free their minds from the clutter of obvious hypotheses and consider the data from a creative angle to reveal new clues and possibilities (Franklin 2012; Sharry et al. 2012). As Poe tells us in "The Purloined Letter," the best place to hide anything is where everyone can see it. Making the shift from problem-focused conversations to solution-focused conversations can be very difficult given the fact that the bulk of training in medical school and residency focuses on problem detection and diagnosis. Physicians are taught the importance of looking for and analyzing problems and skillfully pinpointing what is wrong in patients' lives. Case discussions with colleagues become centered on elaborate exposures of patient symptoms and problems. In medical school, formulations center on masterfully framing an interpretation or diagnosis. When learning solution-focused therapy, clinicians become interested in the reverse process. What if, instead of putting all this time and effort into understanding and categorizing symptoms and problems, clinicians instead channeled more of their energy and training into pinpointing and "diagnosing" patient strengths (Sharry et al. 2012)? What if physicians became skilled at uncovering and exploring differences that lead to positive change? What if, instead of masterfully framing a diagnosis, they focus attention on uncovering hidden potentials and positive differences that patients are already accomplishing, but as yet are unaware of? What if more time were spent on framing compliments that were genuine and well timed, inspiring patients to move forward in their lives? This is in essence the reorientation on which solution-focused therapy is based.

With the continual rise of medical costs and seemingly endless increasing demands on a clinician's time, it is essential that clinicians learn how to create conversations that are therapeutic, brief, and cost-effective. Physicians acquire many skills and interventions that they bring to the therapeutic encounter. Many of these treatments and interventions are costly, adding to this era's ever-increasing medical costs: technical procedures, surgeries, pharmacology, X-rays, laboratory tests, MRIs, CT scans, ECGs, and EEGs to name a few. The expertise of co-creating conversations with patients is powerful, cost-effective, and often greatly underappreciated. Physicians learn in medical school that a good history can lead to an accurate diagnosis as much as 95% of the time. For clinicians, and for therapists in particular, conversations are the primary tool used for assessment and treatment. Much as a surgeon is required to learn anatomy, anesthesia, the use of a scalpel, and broad technical expertise in order to perform successful surgery, performing solution-focused therapy requires tremendous skill, expertise, and practice. The surgeon maneuvers the scalpel. The solution-focused clinician utilizes language and carefully constructed questions as a metaphorical scalpel.

Becoming a solution-focused clinician can be learned, much as a new language is acquired. For students in training who begin seeing patients for therapy, the task is often daunting and filled with anxiety. Articles, readings, and lectures frequently focus on theories but do little to teach students how to do therapy. It is rare that students watch live therapy sessions, are taught the meticulous details of how to construct and time useful questions, or are instructed in detail what to pay attention to and what to ignore. This book aims to teach the skills that one needs to become an expert in using solution-focused conversational skills, identifying and amplifying positive patient factors, co-creating solution-focused conversations that simultaneously strengthen the therapeutic alliance, and guiding patients toward their goals and best hopes for their desired future. Tables 1–1 and 1–2 compare problem-focused and solution-focused "lenses" for viewing clinical work.

TABLE 1–1.	Clinician using a problem-focused lens

- Elicits and amplifies symptoms in order to uncover the root problem
- Makes a diagnosis based on symptoms and pathology
- Attempts to fix the problems and treat the symptoms
- Categorizes problems and applies diagnosis
- Identifies precipitants, predisposing factors, and perpetuating elements of symptoms and problems
- As expert diagnostician, prescribes treatment

TABLE 1–2.	Clinician using a solution-focused lens

- Listens for clues that reveal hidden strengths and resources
- Identifies and amplifies positive differences and as yet unidentified successes
- Inquires who are the most important people in a patient's life
- Assists patients in developing and articulating their best hopes for their preferred future
- Examines how patients have coped and managed despite trauma, mental illness, and disease

LEARNING EXERCISE: SOLUTION-FOCUSED CASE REVIEW

Let's read the following case study. The challenge is to examine this case through a solution-focused lens, closely observing for clues to solutions, hidden strengths, and resources. The reader is invited to think about the following questions:

1. What clues to the solutions are in this description?
2. What questions might you ask to explore these hidden strengths and resources?
3. What compliments could you give to this mother based on only the information presented?

Amy is the mother of four children, ages 4 to 19, two of whom are stepchildren. She brought in Ben, her 12-year-old son, for a second opinion. Amy was referred by another child psychiatrist to clarify whether her son has bipolar disorder and whether his medications are appropriate. At the time of the referral, things were in a rapid state of deterioration for Ben. His mother was concerned about his current treatment and whether there was something else she could do to help her son. Ben was being treated for attention-deficit/hyperactivity disorder (ADHD) and bipolar disorder. He had had trials of multiple medications in the past with only moderate success. These medications included methylphenidate (tried in three formulations: Metadate, Ritalin, and Concerta) as well as aripiprazole (Abilify), sertraline (Zoloft), and risperidone (Risperdal). He has been taking aripiprazole and Metadate for the past year. The school was calling frequently, and he was being suspended two or three times a week. He had missed several homework assignments and was failing three subjects despite receiving services through an Individualized Education Program (IEP). Amy recently got back together with her husband, who in the past was addicted to drugs and abusive toward both Amy and her children. Amy had depression and a history of being a target of domestic abuse by several past partners. Ben's biological father reportedly had bipolar disorder and a substance use disorder and was living in a shelter. As a result, Ben rarely saw his father. His mother expressed her frustration with Ben's treatment progress and wanted to get some answers regarding his "crazy and out-of-control behavior." She described these behaviors as lasting up to 2 hours, leaving them both feeling frustrated and exhausted. During these episodes, he would often make statements that he wanted to kill himself and would say very angry and hurtful things to his mother, further increasing her emotional stress.

Let's begin by trying to identify as many strengths and compliments as possible based only on what was described in this case description.

1. Amy has four children, a relatively large family. It takes considerable skill to parent such a large family, especially accounting for a blended family including two stepchildren. How has she managed this? What skills does she have to cope with these challenges? What has she learned from this? What skills has she found most useful? Who has been most helpful for her? What aspects of parenting does she think she performs well?

2. The referral only mentions problems with this child. Perhaps her other children are doing well in school or in other places. It is worth exploring what her other children are doing and what has helped them do well. This may help reveal what aspects of parenting are helpful. Could some of these skills be helpful for Ben?

3. Amy has worked hard to get Ben services over a long time and is willing to come for a second opinion. She has stuck with Ben and had not given up on him. What has helped her to persevere and not give up on her son? Where has she gotten the strength to do this? It is not easy accessing child psychiatry services and following up with all these appointments. How has she done this?

4. Ben is getting suspended two to three times a week. How is he managing to stay out of trouble on the other days? His outbursts last up to 2 hours; how does he eventually calm down? She reports that he verbally fights. What does he do instead of becoming physically aggres-

sive? If he does get aggressive, how does he eventually stop? Ben states he wants to kill himself. What has stopped him from acting on this? What are his reasons for living? Ben is on an IEP. These are difficult to get into place. How did his mother manage to advocate for these services for Ben? What has been most helpful from these services? He is failing three subjects. What subjects is he passing and doing better in? How is he able to do this?

5. He has been taking Abilify and Metadate for the past year. How have these medications been helpful? On a scale of 1–10, with 10 being a magic pill and 1 being they are not helpful, how helpful are his medications? What do Ben and his mother do that helps the medications work?

6. Despite his father being in a Veterans' shelter, his mother finds a way for Ben to visit his father at least sometimes. This must be very difficult. How has she been able to do this?

7. Amy has gotten out of several abusive relationships. How has she done this? Where has she found the strength to do this? Has anyone helped her do this? How has she coped with these difficulties and managed given the complexity and difficulties of her problems? Her answers may reveal a desire to better herself and her family. She must have a "good reason" to get back together with her husband given the difficulties she described. What does she know about herself and her husband that she decided to have him come back home? What would she say her children would notice that would tell her things are better this time?

8. Amy has had contact with treatment providers for a long time. What has she found most helpful from her treatment providers? What has been most helpful from her treatment providers in the past?

Reviewing a case in this way can lead to a change in perception and attitude on the part of the child, the mother, and the clinician. When questions are asked and explored in this way, it communicates an accepting and empathic attitude promoting engagement while at the same time identifying and amplifying positive patient factors necessary to promote change. The clinician, child, and family are all strengthened by this conversation.

Core Assumptions of the Solution-Focused Clinician

All therapists, regardless of their approach, have certain attitudes and philosophies that affect how they do treatment. When clinicians are talking with patients, the clinicians' beliefs, attitudes, and underlying assumptions about what they believe to be helpful for patients influence how and what they listen for, what they choose to ask about, and what they ignore. The solution-focused clinician assumes that patients are competent until proven otherwise and that they have the necessary resources to live a more satisfying life. Maintaining an attitude of belief in the strengths and capabilities of patients is a critical skill in learning solution-focused therapy. This belief is conveyed through the use of questions and through verbal and nonverbal skills. A fundamental tenet for the solution-focused clinician is a belief in the patient's competence (Berg 2000). Conversations and questions are generated with an attitude that focuses on patient's abilities and strengths. The questions that are asked, their timing, the aspects of conversation that are amplified, and specific choices of language all are used to attempt to magnify the capabilities of patients. The solution-focused clinician remains mindful when listening to patients in order to identify these qualities, amplify positive differences, and uncover as yet undiscovered strengths and resources.

Table 1–3 lists the core solution-focused assumptions.

Several principles are important when the clinician is learning how to integrate core solution-focused assumptions into the conversation. Acknowledging these assumptions out loud with children and parents expresses compelling truths that they rarely hear and that are very powerful. Asking what children appreciate most about their parents is rarely if ever done and is extremely valuable in identifying and uncovering relational strengths between the child and parent. Commenting to parents about how much they love their child, how hard they work for their child, and how persistently they do not give up on their child despite all the challenges highlights parental competencies within the core assumptions. Noticing with parents and children together how proud the parent is of the child's potential, strengths, and accomplishments compliments both the child and parent. Parents love to hear good things about their child, and children want their parents to feel proud of them.

Questions are of the essence.

"I never learn anything talking. I only learn things when I ask questions."
—Lou Holtz, *The New York Times*

Useful questions that are well timed are critical in performing effective therapy with patients. Positive generative questions direct attention and action in specific directions and are powerful therapeutic tools. Generative questions challenge limiting beliefs and assumptions, create fresh insights, and help patients create new meanings while amplifying positive qualities, all of which helps patients move toward their goals (Kelm 2005). People learn, grow, and develop in the areas that are focused on. Solution-focused

TABLE 1–3. Core solution-focused assumptions

Parents

Unless the contrary is proven, a solution-focused clinician believes that all parents have a need to...

1. Be proud of their child
2. Know that their child has the potential to succeed in life
3. See their child happy and healthy
4. Have a good relationship with their child
5. Have a positive influence on their child
6. Hear good news about their child and what their child is good at
7. Give their child a good education and a good chance at success
8. See their child's future as better than theirs
9. Be hopeful about their child
10. Be good parents
11. Have their child experience good friends and healthy relationships
12. Trust their child
13. Provide a healthy and happy home for their child
14. Have fun with their child
15. Be a good role model for their child
16. Have their child contribute to the world around them

Children

Unless the contrary is proven, a solution-focused clinician believes that all children have a need to...

1. Have their parents be proud of them
2. Hear good things about themselves from their parents
3. Feel appreciated by their parents and family
4. Be nurtured and loved by their parents
5. Feel safe and protected
6. Feel cared for physically and emotionally
7. Please their parents and other adults
8. Be trusted by their parents
9. Be accepted as part of a social group
10. Feel they are normal
11. Feel accepted and experience a sense of belonging by their peers

TABLE 1–3.   Core solution-focused assumptions *(continued)*

Children *(continued)*

12. Be active and involved in activities with others

13. Learn new skills

14. Be surprised and surprise others

15. Make choices when given an opportunity

16. Be appreciated for making the right choices

17. Have responsibilities

18. Make a difference for someone else

19. Be valued as a unique individual with special talents, gifts, and dreams

20. Feel a sense of belonging to their family, school, and peer group

Families

Unless the contrary is proven, a solution-focused clinician believes that family members have a need to…

1. Have loving and positive relationships among family members

2. Be listened to and listen to each other

3. Be respected and affirmed by one another

4. Feel they are contributing members of the family

5. Care about the well being of each member of the family

6. Be appreciated and affirmed by one another

7. Give and receive encouragement

8. Recognize and accept differences among each family member

9. Feel accepted through all the normal and natural phases of life

10. Reinforce positive possibilities in each member

11. Recognize each other's unique talents, gifts, abilities, and dreams

12. Help each other recognize their gifts and apply them in making a positive contribution

13. Provide boundaries based on healthy values. Boundaries are agreements among family members that specify what actions are appropriate (e.g., bedtimes, kind language, respect, doing homework, helping clean up)

14. Live in a trusting and safe environment

15. Participate in creating a safe and mutually supportive environment within which family members can care for one another

16. Share stories together

17. Share their dreams with each other

TABLE 1–3.   Core solution-focused assumptions *(continued)*

Families *(continued)*

18. Have a strong sense of belonging with each other

19. Support each other in times of need, loss, tragedy, and celebration

20. Feel respected and validated when expressing feelings, thoughts, dreams, and challenges

21. Have fun together

22. Share in rituals and traditions to celebrate their unique culture

23. Live in a peaceful home where there is mutual love, support, and respect for each other

24. Make a difference for each other, the family, and the community

25. Celebrate special occasions together

---

questions ask about strengths and positive differences, allowing patients to expand their perceptions and ideas of what they need to do in order to live a more satisfying life. When parents ask about the problems their children experience at school, they are conveying to their children that they care about these problems, and the parents, along with their children, become experts in these areas. When parents ask their children about the most exciting or inspiring new idea they heard in school, what they did today that they are most pleased about, and what they did to make themselves or others happy, they convey that they value discovering exciting and inspiring new ideas, and together they become wise and knowledgeable in these areas. The questions asked are fateful. They set the agenda for learning, growth, relational development, and hope. People who are asked to talk about their problems, weaknesses, or fears tend to re-create those experiences in their minds and hearts, and this often deters the generation of ideas that will help them solve their problems. When people are asked positive questions, such as to name something they did today that they are pleased about, the moments parents and children enjoy together, the times when they have been at their best, the best thing that happened in a day, or the things that keep a smile on their face, they are helped to identify positive experiences they have already had (Kelm 2005).

Many of the solution-focused questions ask whether behaviors, feelings, or situations are different from usual. In order for change to happen and therapy to be effective, differences must occur. Dialogs are paused when the clinician identifies any potential positive difference. If these differences are confirmed with the patient, further inquiry expands on how these differences are helpful and what the patient has done to make them occur. In this way the conversation uncovers times when patients have already experienced success, increasing their self-efficacy and hope. (More about how to identify and amplify positive differences will come in Chapter 2, "Beginning With Strengths and Resources.") Solution-focused questions inquire about creative possibilities for an ideal future. The more vivid and detailed a person's dream is for the future, the more likely it is that the person will achieve it. In this model, solutions that a patient creates have more to do with what the person's best hopes are for the preferred future, who the most important people are in his or her life, and what successes the person has already accomplished but is as yet unaware of.

The solution-focused clinician is a conversational artist. Language and questions that focus on success create more success. Far from serving the objective purpose of merely gathering data, the questions clinicians raise with their patients influence and change their thinking about themselves (Berg and De Jong 1996). Solutions for patients are not scientific puzzles to be solved by practitioners, but rather changes in perception, patterns of interacting and living, and meanings that are co-constructed within the patients' frame of reference (de Shazer and Berg 1992). In this model of therapy, both the patient and the clinician are experts, but in different arenas. Patients are the experts on their own problems, who and what is most important to them, their best hopes for their preferred future, and the strengths and resources that they can draw on to produce the changes they desire. The solution-focused clinician is also an expert, but the clinician's expertise lies in the art of how to facilitate and co-create a conversation that amplifies and details what a patient's best hopes are, identifies and amplifies successes a patient is as yet unaware of, and facilitates what the patient needs to do as the next steps to achieve his or her goals. This requires effective interviewing skills.

Interviewing is a unique type of conversation that is co-created with patients and guided by the interviewer. Effective interviewing involves learning and integrating many skills, both verbal and nonverbal. Verbal skills include knowing how to formulate and ask useful questions, when to ask questions, and when to pause the conversation in order to amplify certain aspects of the dialog. Verbal skills also include knowing what to ignore and when to ignore it while talking with patients. Nonverbal skills include modulation of voice tone, body posture, and facial expression. Masterful interviewing skills are a powerful intervention that can directly influence how patients view both their problems and the solutions to their problems (Okun 1997). Learning solution-focused therapy requires meticulous and "surgical" skill when it comes to timing questions and formulating questions. Useful questions well timed are therapeutic powerhouses. For the solution-focused clinician, there are no neutral questions.

Guiding the conversation through the use of questions conveys several important things to patients. Questions convey an inherent belief in the capacity of patients and communicate a genuine curiosity to learn about their perspective without imposing the clinician's own preconceived ideas, assumptions, or judgments. Formulating and asking good questions requires intense and focused listening on the part of the clinician, and when done well it creates an almost meditative experience for both the interviewee and the interviewer. Well-formulated questions incorporate a patient's exact words or paraphrase those words within the question. Clarifying with patients exactly what they mean by the specific words they use communicates a genuine curiosity about and interest in understanding their perspective, further validating their unique experience. When a patient's exact words are used within a solution-focused question, the conversation moves beyond reflective listening (which in essence is parroting back what the patient says). Questions guide the dialog toward constructive change that a patient will be required to make to meet desired goals.

Mastering fluency in the core solution-focused questions requires some memorization and practice, much as proficiency and expertise must be attained when one is learning a new language or learning diagnostic categories and symptom constellations. Table 1–4 presents the core solution-focused questions. Throughout this book, these questions will be repeated, reviewed, and elaborated on with the hope that the reader can become fluent in co-creating solution-focused conversations with client patients and families.

Let's look at a brief example in order to demonstrate how some of these questions are used in creating conversations with patients. Notice that each question has a purpose and is carefully formulated based on the patient's responses. Pay attention to how negative statements are changed to positive goals. Pay attention to how the clinician listens closely for any opportunities to compliment the patient and how these opportunities are amplified with the patient. All these skills and more will be exemplified throughout this book with the hope that by the end, you will learn how to become both competent and confident in practicing solution-focused conversational techniques.

Case Illustration: Using Questions in Conversation With a Patient

Beth is an 18-year-old woman who has suffered significant loss and trauma. Her father died by suicide when she was only 14 years old, and she experienced emotional abuse as well as witnessing domestic violence, a high degree of parental conflict, and divorce. She had been diagnosed with a non-verbal learning disorder as well as depression and executive functioning difficulties.

TABLE 1–4.	**Core solution-focused questions**

Beginning with strengths

- What are you good at and do you enjoy doing?
- How did you become good at this?
- What else are you good at or do you enjoy?
- What do you know about your child that tells you they will succeed in life?
- What else do you know about them that tells you they will succeed in life?
- Where did they get this potential?

Exploring VIPs

- Who are the most important people in your life? (VIPs)
- Who else are the most important people in your life?
- What do you most appreciate about them?
- What else do you appreciate about them?
- Whose idea was it that you come here?
- Who was worried about you that thought coming here would be helpful for you?
- What would tell them that you no longer need to be here for treatment?

Goal negotiation (chief complaint)

- How can I be most helpful for you today so that this meeting is worthwhile?
- What are your best hopes for this meeting?
- What have you tried to do that has been helpful for you?
- What else have you tried that has helped?

Identification and amplification of positive differences

- Was this different for you?
- How was it different for you?
- Was it helpful for you?
- How was it helpful for you?
- How did you do it?
- How else did you do it?
- Were things different between you and others because of this?
- How were things different between you and your VIPs/others?
- On a scale of 1–10, where 10 is you are confident you could do this again and 1 is the opposite, where would you say you are now?
- What makes it not lower?

TABLE 1–4.   Core solution-focused questions *(continued)*

Identification and amplification of positive differences

- What else makes it not lower?
- What would it take to raise it by one point?

Follow-up sessions

- What is better since I last saw you?
- What else is better?
- What is better between you and your VIPs since we last met?
- What would your VIPs say is better?
- What else would they say is better?
- How could I be most helpful for you today so that this meeting is worthwhile for you?
- What are your best hopes for the meeting today?

Miracle question and amplification

- Suppose after you go to bed and fall asleep tonight, a miracle happens. This miracle happens when you are sleeping. The miracle is that all the problems and worries that brought you in to see me today are gone. It is as if when you woke up it was a "10 miracle day," but because you were asleep when the miracle happened you were not aware that it occurred. When you wake up in the morning, as you are lying in bed and going through your day, what would tell you that this miracle has happened?
- What would you notice you would be doing differently when this miracle has happened?
- What else would you be doing?
- What would your VIPs notice you doing when this miracle happens?
- What else would your VIPs notice you doing?
- What would be different between you and your VIPs when this miracle happens?
- What else would be different between you and your VIPs?
- Supposing 10 is the day after the miracle and 1 is the opposite, where would you say things are now?
- What makes it not lower?
- What else makes it not lower?
- What would make it one point higher?
- Supposing we asked your VIPs where would they rate things from 1–10 for you in regards to your miracle day?

TABLE 1–4.   **Core solution-focused questions** *(continued)*

Coping questions

- How have you coped with this?
- How have you managed?
- Where do you get your strength?
- On a scale of 1–10, where 10 is you are satisfied with how you are coping and 1 is the opposite, where would you say you are now?
- What makes it not lower?
- What else makes it not lower?
- What would it take to raise it by one point?
- Where would your VIPs rate how you are coping on a scale of 1–10?
- What do you need?
- What else do you need?

Yes-set confirmation responses

- Of course that must be very difficult "for you."
- That must be so frustrating "for you."
- That must really stink "for you."

Questions that amplify ambivalence

- You must have a "good reason" to (insert any seemingly harmful behaviors—using drugs, fighting, cutting, etc.)
- How is it helpful "for you" to (insert any seemingly harmful behaviors—using drugs, yelling, hitting, etc.)?
- How else is it helpful for you?
- On a scale of 1–10, how helpful is this behavior for you?
- On a scale of 1–10, how unhelpful is this behavior for you?
- On a scale of 1–10, how helpful would your VIPs say this behavior is for you?
- On a scale of 1–10, how unhelpful would your VIPs say this behavior is for you?
- What makes the number not lower?

Reframing negative statements

- What would you do instead of (fill in the blank for any unhelpful behaviors)?
- What else would you do instead?

Scaling questions

- On a scale of 1–10, where 10 is you are very confident in your ability to reach your goals and 1 is the opposite, where would you rate things now?
- On a scale of 1–10, how would you rate things between you and your VIPs?

TABLE 1–4.   Core solution-focused questions *(continued)*

Scaling questions *(continued)*

- On a scale of 1–10, how would you rate your progress toward your goals?
- On a scale of 1–10, where 10 is you are satisfied that your problem is solved and 1 is the opposite, where would you say things are now?
- What makes it not lower?
- What would it take to raise it by one point?
- On a scale of 1–10, where 10 is you are confident you can keep yourself safe and 1 is the opposite, where would you say you are now?
- What makes it not lower?
- What else makes it not lower?
- What would it take to raise it by one point?
- What number would you need to go to the hospital or call for help?
- How confident are your VIPs that you can keep yourself safe?
- How confident are you that you can calm down/ listen/ stay sober/ remain calm as a parent from 1–10?
- What makes it not lower?
- What else makes it not lower?
- Supposing 10 is the medication is helping like a magic pill, and 1 is the opposite, how helpful is the medication for you?

The following is an excerpt taken from a follow-up session with Beth.

ANNE: What's been better since the last time we met?
　　Notice that the first question asked is "What is better?" This question imme-diately homes in on looking for positive differences and successes.
BETH *(pause)*: Well, I've made a little bit of progress.
ANNE: What progress have you made?
　　Notice how the clinician chooses her exact word, "progress," within the question to highlight this positive difference, creating a shared dialect with the patient.
BETH: I've checked the university's Web site and what credits I need in or-der to apply for community college courses.
ANNE: Is that different that you were able to do all this?
　　Difference questions are extremely valuable. Asking whether a behavior, atti-tude, or relationship is different obtains confirmation respectfully from pa-tients as to whether they have noticed this, and it is the first step toward amplifying differences. More "yes" responses garnered within a conversation build the strength of the therapeutic alliance as agreement is noted. In order for change to occur, something different needs to happen. When a positive difference is observed, a success has already occurred, and this is critical to magnify.

BETH: Yes, I guess it is.

It is very helpful to take the time to get "yes" responses. These yes responses sustain the conversational flow of agreement and are essential to maintain a collaborative and strong treatment alliance.

ANNE: How was this different?

This question garners the problem and symptoms while simultaneously creating a narrative of strength.

BETH: I usually just can't get myself to call and end up staying up late playing my video games and sleeping the day away.

ANNE: Was it helpful for you to do this?

This question is another way to obtain a "yes" confirmation while respectfully asking whether the patient thinks this difference was helpful.

BETH: Yes.

ANNE: How was it helpful for you?

This question obtains another "yes" response confirming and validating the patient's perspective that this behavior was in fact helpful for her.

BETH: It gave me some hope that maybe I can get into a college.

ANNE: How have you been able to do this?

This question further magnifies the positive difference by encouraging the patient to think about what she "did" to accomplish this difference. It is a way to indirectly compliment patients and highlight their accomplishments while helping them realize the behavior they actually engaged in to accomplish this task. When the patient has already had a success and this is amplified, it gives her much more confidence that she can do this again and in so doing increases her self-efficacy.

BETH: I'm trying to think less and act more.

ANNE: Is that different that you were able to think less and act more?

Another "Is it different?" question highlights another potential positive difference. Notice how the patient's exact words "think less and act more" are incorporated within the question. Another round of questions to amplify this difference will follow: How was it different? Was it helpful? How was it helpful? How did you do it?

BETH: Yes, it was.

Another "yes" confirmation.

ANNE: How was it different?

The same lines of questions that amplify this difference are repeated.

BETH: I usually just do the most comfortable thing, which is to play my video games. This time I went to bed at a reasonable time and woke up and looked up on the computer what I needed to do in order to enroll in a community college.

ANNE: That must have been very difficult for you and taken a lot of work.

It is crucial to acknowledge how difficult and how much work these differences in behaviors are to accomplish for patients. Adding the words "for you" at the end of statements provides empathy and validation, while giving them a face-saving tool should they not be able to accomplish the task.

BETH: Yes.

Another "yes" response confirming that my validation of her feelings was correct. The brief time it takes to confirm this emotional experience goes a long way toward sustaining and strengthening the therapeutic alliance.

ANNE: Was it helpful for you to think less and act more?

This question persists in the line of questions that amplify positive differences she is making, while meticulously persevering in using the patient's exact words within the solution-focused question.

BETH: Yes, it was.

Another "yes" response taking the time to confirm the patient's experience.

ANNE: How was it helpful?

This question continues to amplify the positive difference.

BETH: I was able to think about what I want for my future and that I don't want to lose my relationship with my boyfriend. He is going to college and I think if I don't do more he may not want to stay with me.

ANNE: That must be very difficult for you to think about losing your boyfriend. How were you able to think less and act more?

Validating her response by adding a "for you" statement regarding the concerns she has about her boyfriend is followed by a solution-focused question, asking how did you do it, further detailing her success.

BETH: I think it's fear.

ANNE: Fear? What do you mean by fear?

Becoming solution focused requires careful attention to the exact words patients use. Asking patients what they mean by the particular words they choose maintains the patient as expert and facilitates a curious and nonassuming tone, enhancing treatment engagement through the creation of a shared dialect.

BETH: I don't want to be thrown out of the house or be a burden to my family. It scares me to be dependent on others and not be productive.

ANNE: That must be scary for you. What do you want instead of feeling like a burden to your family?

When patients talk about painful and troubling thoughts, it is helpful to tag on the words "for you" at the end of a statement. This is a practical way to validate their experience and maintain agreement, guiding the conversation toward positive "doable" goals.

BETH: I would be living independently, getting a job, and going to school.

ANNE: On a scale of 1–10, where 10 is you are very confident in your ability to move toward becoming independent and 1 is the opposite, where would you rate things now?

Scaling aspects of the conversations helps patients articulate and clarify their goals. This question can then be used in two directions. Asking what makes the number not lower uncovers additional successes and hope.

BETH: It is a 4.

ANNE: What makes it not lower than a 4?

BETH: I'm getting to bed earlier and making an effort to try and call the colleges to find out what courses I need to take.

ANNE: What else makes it not lower?

Asking "What else?" digs for further details of success.

BETH: I'm trying to look for jobs and have been going on Craigslist every day.

ANNE: That's a lot you are doing. What do you suppose would make that number go up to a 5? Not all the way to a 10, just a bit higher?

Bridging a direct compliment about how hard she is working with a scaling question helps negotiate small, doable goals.

BETH: I would actually begin to fill out a college application.

ANNE: That's a good next step, and may be difficult to do. I am wondering how confident you are on a scale of 1–10 that you could begin to fill out a college application?

Scaling a patient's confidence is a good way to assess motivation and is quick and easy to ask. Acknowledging that all steps are hard work appreciates with patients the challenges at hand in making behavioral changes.

BETH: I would say about a 6.

As can be seen from this vignette, every solution-focused question was meticulously formulated and stemmed from the direct response of the patient. Questioning in this way requires intense listening and concentration on the part of the clinician. These questions and techniques assist patients in creating narratives that help them rigorously describe their goals and best hopes for their desired future, while uncovering the necessary resources to accomplish their goals. The following chapters will further exemplify this approach, beginning with an exploration of strengths and resources.

KEY POINTS

- Solution building differs from problem solving.
- In the solution-focused approach, a patient's solutions are not necessarily directly related to any problem identified by either the patient or the therapist.
- The therapeutic focus is on the patient's desired future rather than on past problems or current conflicts.
- Patients are encouraged to increase the frequency of useful behaviors.
- This approach assumes that patients are competent until proven otherwise and have the necessary resources to live a more satisfying life.
- Language and questions that focus on success create more success.
- Solutions for patients are not scientific puzzles to be solved by practitioners, but rather changes in perception.
- Conversations are co-constructed within the patient's frame of reference.
- Both the patient and the clinician are the experts, but in different arenas. Clients are the experts on their problems, strengths, and best hopes for their future. The clinician is the expert at noticing what works, identifying strengths and resources, and guiding the conversation through the useful questions.
- The conversational skills required to help patients build solutions are different from those needed to diagnose problems.

References

Berg IK: Family Based Services: A Solution-Focused Approach. New York, WW Norton, 1994

Berg IK: Working Assumptions. Milwaukee, WI, BFTC Press, 2000

Berg IK, De Jong P: Solution-building conversations: co-constructing a sense of competence with clients. Families in Society 77:376–391, 1996

Berg IK, Miller SD: Working With the Problem Drinker: A Solution-Focused Approach. New York, WW Norton, 1992

Bernes K: The Elements of Effective Counselling. University of Lethbridge, 2005. Available at: https://www.uleth.ca/dspace/bitstream/handle/10133/1167/The%20Elements%20of%20Effective%20Counselling_NATCON.pdf?sequence=1. Accessed February 15, 2013.

De Jong P, Berg IK: Interviewing for Solutions. Belmont, CA, Thomson Brooks/Cole Publishing, 1998

de Shazer S: Keys to Solution in Brief Therapy. New York, WW Norton, 1985

de Shazer S: Clues: Investigating Solutions in Brief Therapy. New York, NY, WW Norton, 1988

de Shazer S, Berg IK: Doing therapy: a post-structural re-vision. Journal of Marital and Family Therapy 18:71–81, 1992

de Shazer S, Berg IK: "What works?" Remarks on research aspects of solution-focused brief therapy. Journal of Family Therapy 19:121–124, 1997

de Shazer S, Berg IK, Lipchik E, et al: Brief therapy: focused solution development. Fam Process 25:207–221, 1986

Dolan YM: Resolving Sexual Abuse: Solution-Focused Therapy and Ericksonian Hypnosis for Adult Survivors. New York, WW Norton, 1991

Erickson MH: Further clinical techniques of hypnosis: utilization techniques. 1959. Am J Clin Hypn 51:341–362, 2009a

Erickson MH: Naturalistic techniques of hypnosis. 1958. Am J Clin Hypn 51:333–340, 2009b

Franklin C: Solution-Focused Brief Therapy: A Handbook of Evidence-Based Practice. New York, Oxford University Press, 2012

Franklin C, Moore K, Hopson L: Effectiveness of solution-focused brief therapy in a school setting. Children and Schools 30:15–26, 2008

Furman B, Ahola T: Solution Talk: Hosting Therapeutic Conversations. New York, WW Norton, 1992

Holyoake D, Golding E: Multiculturalism and solution-focused psychotherapy: an exploration of the nonexpert role. Asia Pacific Journal of Counselling and Psychotherapy 3:72–81, 2012

Hoyt MF, Berg IK: Solution-focused couple therapy: helping clients construct self-fulfilling realities, in The Handbook of Constructive Therapies: Innovative Approaches From Leading Practitioners. Edited by Hoyt MF. San Francisco, CA, Jossey-Bass, 1998, pp. 314–340

Iveson C, George E, Ratner H: Brief Coaching: A Solution Focused Approach. New York, Routledge/Taylor & Francis Group, 2012

Kelly MS, Bluestone-Miller R: Working on What Works (WOWW): coaching teachers to do more of what's working. Children and Schools 31:35–38, 2009

Kelm JB: Appreciative Living: The Principles of Appreciative Inquiry in Personal Life. Wake Forest, NC, Venet Publishers, 2005

Kim JS, Smock S, Trepper TS, et al: Is solution-focused brief therapy evidence-based? Families in Society 91:300–306, 2010

Lambert MJ: Psychotherapy outcome and quality improvement: introduction to the special section on patient-focused research. J Consult Clin Psychol 69:147–149, 2001

Lambert MJ: Early response in psychotherapy: further evidence for the importance of common factors rather than "placebo effects." J Clin Psychol 61:855–869, 2005

Lambert MJ, Barley DE: Research summary on the therapeutic relationship and psychotherapy outcome. Psychotherapy: Theory, Research, Practice, Training 38:357–361, 2001

Lee Duckworth A, Steen TA, Seligman ME: Positive psychology in clinical practice. Annu Rev Clin Psychol 1:629–651, 2005

Metcalf L: Solution Focused Group Therapy: Ideas for Groups in Private Practice, Schools, Agencies, and Treatment Programs. New York, Free Press, 1998

Nelson TS: Solution-focused brief couple therapy, in Case Studies in Couples Therapy: Theory-Based Approaches. Edited by Carson DK, Casado-Kehoe M. New York, Routledge/Taylor & Francis Group, 2011, pp 275–287

Okun BF: Effective Helping: Interviewing and Counseling Techniques. Pacific Grove, CA, Brooks/Cole Publishing, 1997

Pichot T, Smock SA: Solution-Focused Substance Abuse Treatment. New York, Routledge/Taylor & Francis Group, 2009

Roeden JM, Bannink FP, Maaskant MA, et al: Solution-focused brief therapy with persons with intellectual disabilities. Journal of Policy and Practice in Intellectual Disabilities 6:253–259, 2009

Rogers CR: Carl Rogers on the development of the person-centered approach. Person-Centered Review 1:257–259, 1986

Selekman MD: Solution-Focused Therapy With Children: Harnessing Family Strengths for Systemic Change. New York, Guilford, 1997

Selekman MD: Integrative, solution-oriented approaches with self-harming adolescents, in The School Practitioner's Concise Companion to Health and Well-Being. Edited by Franklin C, Harris MB, Allen-Meares P. New York, Oxford University Press, 2008, pp 109–118

Sell NK: Review of preventing suicide: the solution focused approach. J Dev Behav Pediatr 32:17, 2011

Sharry J, Madden B, Darmody M: Becoming a Solution Detective: A Strengths-Based Guide to Brief Therapy, 2nd Edition. New York, Routledge/Taylor & Francis Group, 2012

Simon JK: Solution Focused Practice in End-of-Life and Grief Counseling. New York, Springer, 2010

Stith SM, McCollum EE, Rosen KH: Domestic violence-focused couples therapy within a solution-focused framework, in Couples Therapy for Domestic Violence: Finding Safe Solutions. Edited by Stith SM, McCollum EE, Rosen KH. Washington, DC, American Psychological Association, 2011, pp 31–42

Tews-Kozlowski R: Solution-focused therapy with military couples, in Handbook of Counseling Military Couples. Edited by Moore BA. New York, Routledge/Taylor & Francis Group, 2012, pp 53–87

Trepper TS, Dolan Y, McCollum EE, et al: Steve de Shazer and the future of solution-focused therapy. J Marital Fam Ther 32:133–139, 2006

Watzlawick P, Fisch R, Andolfi M, et al: Strategic and structural approaches, in *What Is Psychotherapy? Contemporary Perspectives.* Edited by Zeig JK, Munion WM, San Francisco, CA, Jossey-Bass, 1990, pp 266–305

Ziegler P, Hiller T: Solution-focused therapy with couples, in *Handbook of Solution-Focused Brief Therapy: Clinical Applications.* Edited by Nelson TS, Thomas FN. New York, Haworth, 2007, pp 91–115

CHAPTER 2

Beginning With Strengths and Resources

The Therapeutic Alliance

At the heart of all therapy lies the human relationship. The therapeutic alliance with our patients is the base from which all therapy begins, and building an alliance is a critical skill to learn in caring for others. Unless patients believe that the clinician is on their side and is there to help them, progress in treatment is difficult if not impossible. Across all forms of therapy, the therapeutic relationship is extremely important in influencing a positive outcome. Knowing how to navigate the complexities and nuances of establishing a therapeutic alliance, especially in the initial encounter, is arguably one of the most important skills for a therapist to master (Cheng 2007). For a clinician working with children and families, gaining mastery at building simultaneous alliances with dyads, parents, children, adolescents, and others important in a patient's life can be a demanding and even a formidable task. The challenge is often further complicated by the need to engage with the myriad outside relationships involved in a child's life, such as negotiating goals with divorced parents in a high-conflict divorce, step-parents, siblings, grandparents, Department of Children and Families (DCF) workers, teachers, primary care physicians, probation officers, and other treatment providers involved in the care of a child. These challenges are particularly intense when adults involved in the care of children are disputing with one another and putting the child in the middle of highly charged and conflict-ridden situations. How can clinicians communicate that they are hearing a parent's litany of problems and concerns about their child, while at the same time not exacerbating how bad the child feels about him- or herself? How can clinicians maintain the alliance of divorced parents who have differing and very strong opinions regarding medication for their child? There are no easy answers in these complex situations, but the solution-focused conversational skills demonstrated in the following chapters can help with what can feel like a Herculean task.

Many factors are associated with achieving a strong therapeutic alliance. Lambert and Barley talk about common factors that contribute most to positive therapeutic outcome (Lambert and Barley 2001). The development and maintenance of the therapeutic relationship is a primary curative component of therapy, providing the context in which specific techniques exert their influence (Lambert and Barley 2001). This chapter will focus on how to uncover, amplify, and diagnose strengths, resources, and positive attributes in a patient's life that are critical for a positive therapeutic outcome, while also strengthening the therapeutic alliance. The chapter will begin with a discussion of problem-free talk.

Starting With Problem-Free Talk

Problem-free talk is an opportunity for patients to talk about parts of their life that are going well and provides them a chance to talk about their strengths and talents that can be drawn upon in the interview (Green et al. 2006). The first step in building a solution-focused conversation from the start is by beginning the conversation with an exploration of the patient's and family's strengths and resources. This is especially important in working with children and adolescents, who almost never want to talk about their problems. It is difficult to have an argument about what people are good at. Building the conversation early around areas of agreement enhances the therapeutic alliance. When engaging in problem-free talk, the clinician is interested in getting to know the child and family as persons with talents, interests, hobbies, positive qualities, hopes, and aspirations (George et al. 2006; Lethem 2002). Problem-free talk is a skilled process. Learning about a person's talents and strengths brings to light the very resources that will be useful for them in overcoming their problems. This conversation is important not only in promoting the treatment alliance and enhancing engagement but also in uncovering potential hidden resources that would otherwise go undetected and could be critical factors that influence patient outcome. It may be tempting to skip this problem-free talk, and some may consider this social chitchat. This is not the case. Skipping problem-free talk puts the clinician at risk of missing crucial resources for the treatment of patients and their families. Focusing only on problems contributes most detrimentally by focusing patients on seeing themselves as ill, limiting their perception of their own strengths—the very strengths they will need to overcome and cope with their problems.

Patients often begin their conversation with a physician immersed in their problem and chief complaint. This is understandable both from the patient's and clinician's perspective. Clinicians are trained to listen to problems and evaluate chief complaints, and people are socialized to talk about their complaints to doctors. This makes it very easy for the physician to see patients only in terms of their presenting problem. Problem-free talk can be likened to an investment banker trying to seize on small investments early that yield a high rate of return. Before withdrawals can be made from a bank, there first need to be adequate funds on account, enough *deposits*. In working with children and adults who have absolutely no desire to give you any of their money (that is, answer your questions and talk with you), it is helpful to first make deposits. These deposits are made through the use of carefully constructed questions that uncover and amplify strengths, resources, and competencies. Another way to think of problem-free talk is as anesthesia for the conversational procedure to follow. Much as a surgeon would not perform surgery without first administering anesthesia, so too a solution-focused clinician would not perform a "surgical conversation" without first taking the time to explore strengths and resources needed to overcome the problem. This is where the traditional medical model has focused less attention. Solution-focused therapy addresses the essential skills and tools to promote a therapeutic alliance in a way in which the medical model used alone has not. It provides complementary skills and reveals therapeutically significant competencies and resources that would otherwise go undetected using only the medical model (De Jong and Berg 1998). This is a particular boon for physicians, who unfortunately are often constrained by insurance limits, time, and the number of patients they are required to see. Using solution-focused interviewing skills can heighten therapeutic effectiveness in a briefer time while simultaneously enhancing the therapeutic alliance (de Shazer et al. 1986). Several questions (Table 2–1) are asked at the beginning of an interview to highlight strengths and resources.

Thanking Patients

Thanking patients is another tool that is helpful in promoting solutions. When people are thanked for things they do or have done, the clinician is conveying that they are already part of the solution. Thanking people and using the words "appreciate" within questions and statements are simple ways to help build engagement. This can be done in high-conflict situations as well. For example, when parents and children are arguing over homework or spouses are arguing over tasks, asking them each to spend a few minutes thanking one another can be a powerful way to change the direction of the

TABLE 2–1.   Initial interview questions that highlight strengths and resources

- What do you enjoy?
- What are you good at?
- How did you learn these skills?
- What else are you good at?
- What else do you enjoy?
- How did you learn these skills?
- How else did you learn them?

conversation in a positive direction. Thanking patients for coming to the session and appreciating how far they have come communicates your appreciation and transmits that they are already part of the solution.

Compliments

Compliments are another tool used frequently and throughout the solution-focused interview (Campbell et al. 1999). Compliments are used in all cultures, and they function to cement social relationships. In this way, they also serve to strengthen the therapeutic alliance. They are not flattery. Flattery is excessive and insincere praise used for the purpose of furthering one's own interests. Compliments are based on honest praise and admiration. There are two main types of compliments, direct and indirect (Berg and De Jong 2005). Direct compliments candidly praise patients on something they reveal. For example, a direct compliment may be commenting with a mother on how she loves her child, will do anything for him, works hard to provide for his needs, and is able to remain calm despite her frustrations. Direct compliments can also include commending patients on their skills at work, at school, or with friends. Indirect compliments take the form of questions (De Jong and Berg 1998). Indirect compliments allow patients to describe their own successes—for example, asking a patient how he or she did something or coped despite the challenges that had to be faced. Many of the questions illustrated in this chapter will demonstrate how to provide indirect compliments.

Learning Exercise 1: Group Compliment Exercise

When patients come in for treatment, they are usually deeply involved in their problems. These problems are the very reasons they are coming to see you. It is easy as a therapist to become immersed in their problems as well, losing sight of the strength they possess. The following is an exercise you can do with another person or a group of people that demonstrates the power of compliments. Ask someone to volunteer to talk about something he or she needs to complain about for 2 minutes. Have the rest of the group listen to the volunteer complainer. They will be asked to comment on what the volunteer has said, but can *only* respond with a compliment. As Yvonne Dolan says, this requires metaphorically growing a third ear (Y. Dolan, personal communication). It is amazing to see how a brief complaint can lead to many compliments, if one only listens for them. Ask the volunteer and group what it felt like to do this exercise. Invariably, the volunteer comments on how much better he or she feels and what a good experience it was. The people acting as therapists are amazed to see how many compliments they could come up with after listening to a series of complaints for only 2 minutes. This exercise is powerful in demonstrating the strength of compliments.

Case Illustration: Problem-Free Talk

Sarah is a 15-year-old girl who was admitted to a drug rehabilitation center after spending 2 weeks in a detoxification facility. She had been suffering from multiple drug addictions, including addictions to nicotine, ecstasy, hydrocodone/acetaminophen (Vicodin), oxycodone, cannabis, and alcohol. Her father was in jail for armed robbery, domestic violence, and drug-related charges. Her mother suffered from posttraumatic stress disorder and depression and had experienced trauma from being in several abusive relationships. As a result, Sarah had witnessed domestic violence throughout her life and had suffered from sexual abuse. I was asked to evaluate Sarah and her mother. I had about 5 minutes to review Sarah's history prior to meeting with her and her mother. It was another hectic day. The staff was anxious to move things along. As usual, there was a whole list of patients to be seen. Where to begin? Let's read some of this interview and see how beginning with problem-free talk can enhance the treatment alliance while simultaneously diagnosing as yet undiscovered resources and strengths.

ANNE (*speaking to Sarah and her mother*): Thank you for taking the time to talk with me. I really appreciate you coming all this way and taking the time to meet. I want to first explain what my role is. I am the child psychiatrist here. I work as part of a team with the other staff, and my hope is that I can be helpful for Sarah and your family. In order to be most helpful, I ask many questions, some of which can be very difficult. I will try my best. Would this be OK with you?

Thanking patients and families for coming and appreciating the time they take to talk with you conveys that they are already part of the solution. I explain my role and obtain their consent for the conversational procedure ahead, and I add that I will try my best. This conveys my hope that they will also try their best. Warning patients of the difficult questions I ask can be especially helpful when they find questions hard to answer. It respectfully appreciates with them the challenges ahead while starting the conversation off in a mutually agreeable direction.

SARAH *and her* MOTHER *both nod yes. Agreement is noted.*

ANNE: Sarah, what are some things that you enjoy or are good at?

I commence the conversation by inquiring about strengths and enjoyment, both areas the adolescent and parent can agree upon. Parents love to hear good things about their children, and children want their parents to feel proud of them. It is difficult to argue about what a child is good at. It is essential that enough conversational time is spent in areas of agreement. Fostering agreement sets the conversational tone and direction of the entire interview.

SARAH: I like poetry and sports.

ANNE: What do you enjoy about poetry?

I gather as many details as I can about every strength.

SARAH: I like writing about things.

ANNE: Have you always liked writing?

I ask if she always has liked writing or if this is something different. If it is different, it may be helpful to ask how it is different and whether it has been helpful.

SARAH: Yes.

ANNE: Is it helpful for you to write poetry?

This question can increase her awareness of a potentially useful skill.

SARAH: Yes.

Confirmation is noted.

ANNE: How has it been helpful for you to write poetry?

I garner further details of how this skill is useful for her, incorporating her words in each question.

SARAH: It helps me get things off my chest.

ANNE: How did you learn to write poetry?

This question is crucial. Asking her how she learned poetry conveys that she has already acquired a skill and that this skill is useful for her, as determined by the previous line of questions. Asking people how they do things is an indirect compliment. When people gain awareness of how they do things, and how these things are helpful for them, they are more able to do more of these things in the future. Inviting patients to detail how they have been able to do things that are helpful for them assists them gently in learning to compliment themselves.

SARAH: I don't know. No one really taught me. It's just something I do.

ANNE: So you learned this on your own? How did you do that?

I provide both a direct and indirect compliment. The direct compliment is that she learned this on her own, and the indirect compliment is asking how she did it. These responses highlight skills she has acquired. Children especially want to learn new skills, and enjoy the challenge of gaining expertise.

SARAH: I don't know. I guess it's just something I do.

ANNE: So you have a lot of creative ability and are really able to use your own initiative and skill to do things that help you feel better.

Providing more direct compliments communicates my belief in her external abilities, writing and poetry, and also her internal abilities, initiative and creativity.

ANNE: What else are you good at?

Asking what else is an extremely simple and useful question. Asking what else is a question that digs for details of strengths and resources, conveying my belief that she has other strengths and competencies that are there, but as yet not revealed. Omitting this question would risk many resources being left unidentified.

SARAH: I don't know.

ANNE (*pause*): I know I ask a lot of hard questions and you may need some time to think about this question (*pause*).

Often children and adolescents answer "I don't know." Calmly pausing and then taking responsibility for the hard questions communicates an appreciation for the hard work it takes to answer them. It also puts the conversational ball back in her court, persisting in the diagnostic pursuit of strengths. Although these questions may appear at first glance simple, that does not mean they are easy. Children and adults alike are rarely directly asked what things they are good at or enjoy. When people pause, it indicates they are being thoughtful about the questions.

SARAH: I was working as a waitress for the past year.

My persistence paid off. She revealed a very important strength.

ANNE: Wow! Even while all this was going on? How did you manage to do this?

I provide a direct compliment, Wow, and an indirect compliment in the form of a question.

SARAH: Well, I had to. How else could I support my drug habit?

At this point it would be easy to get caught up in the problem of her drug habit. Instead, I continue to focus on her strengths, cognizant that it is still very early in the conversation and more conversational deposits need to be made.

ANNE: So you must have been a pretty good waitress to be there for a whole year while also supporting your drug habit? How did you manage?

I provide another direct and indirect compliment. I continue to pursue strengths until she has nothing further positive to add.

SARAH: Yeah, I was pretty good. I had customers who gave me presents and personally requested me. People say I'm pretty friendly.

ANNE: Wow, that's pretty amazing how you managed to not only keep your job, but how well respected you were with the customers. That must have taken a lot of hard work.

I directly compliment more of her inner strengths. Not taking the time to fully assess and uncover all her potential resources would miss potential positive attributes that may be critical for the success of her recovery.

SARAH: I worked for a while, but then I couldn't stand the way I was feeling anymore.

Sarah begins to reveal the problem at her own pace. This is common when enough conversational deposits have been made.

Notice that with conversational deposits came an honest description of Sarah's problems, but the problem description was framed within a narrative that highlighted her accomplishments, came at a pace she felt comfortable with, and in this way promoted the treatment alliance. During this brief initial conversation, she was never asked why she was here. Asking "why" questions, especially when working with children or adolescents, generally results in patients becoming more defensive. Instead, and without delay, the conversation began by questioning the patient about her strengths, resources, and accomplishments. What can be seen from this conversation is that Sarah's problems are revealed, but in a different way than in a traditional problem-focused interview, accentuating her capabilities rather than her deficits. Commencing in this way communicates trust, confidence, and a belief in the patient's potential, strengthening the treatment alliance. This case demonstrates that beginning the conversation with strengths and talents equips the therapist to make conversational deposits early in the interview, highlighting the resources, accomplishments, and achievements with which the patient has already had success, and that so doing further enhances the treatment alliance.

 Video Illustration: Beginning with problem-free talk (2:16)

VIPs: Who Are the Most Important People in Your Patient's Life?

All people live in relationships. Relationships not only are crucial for survival but also are essential resources that help people solve their problems. Uncovering and diagnosing strengths requires assessment of a patient's social context, those individuals and systems that are most important in their life. The important people are called their VIPs (very important people) and are critical to identify early in the conversation. Much as a physician needs a patient's vital signs when determining the person's health, a solution-focused therapist must know who the patient's VIPs are. These relationships will be used throughout the solution-focused interview, so this information is paramount to gather early in the interview. VIPs allow the therapist to assist patients in building solutions from the multiple perspectives of those most important in their life, and these VIPs are often involved in the treatment decisions of patients. There is broad agreement that when a clinician is working with children and those with intellectual and cognitive impairments, assessment requires multiple informants (Kraemer et al. 2003). One important question to consider is how these informants should be selected in order to provide valid assessment information (Kraemer et al. 2003). The solution-focused approach is to ask the patient directly who she thinks are the most important people in her life, thus maintaining the patient as the expert on her social context.

Remember that problems are solved generally in one of two ways. Either the problem is solved or the patient and those most important to the patient

(VIPs) no longer view the behaviors or difficulties as problematic. For problems to be considered solved, the patient's system must be in agreement that there are no significant problems. Learning solution-focused therapy requires broadening the definition of "who" a patient is to include in the unique social context, most importantly the patient's VIPs (Pichot and Smock 2009). The VIPs are the social context in which patients develop their solutions. This means that solution-focused clinicians must ask patients who the most important people in their life are and what they most appreciate about them.

VIPs who are not openly acknowledged are crucial to identify in working with externally motivated (mandated) patients (De Jong and Berg 2001). Asking patients who are the most important people in their life assesses, from their perspective, who will be most helpful in determining when their problems are solved. Two questions are helpful in assessing VIPs in externally motivated patients. The first question is whose idea it was that they come in for treatment. The second is who was "worried" or "concerned" enough about them that they thought coming to treatment would be helpful for them. Asking externally motivated patients what things would tell their VIPs that they no longer need to come for treatment is another useful question that helps patients articulate their goals. These questions often uncover hidden VIPs such as probation officers, DCF workers, or other agencies and people important in the patient's life. For example, adolescents may not mention their probation officer (PO), DCF worker, or judge, but these people are extremely important in determining what they can do, where they can go, what they need to do to get off probation, and whether they can go home to their family.

Asking patients what they most appreciate about their VIPs uncovers strengths and resources related to the patient, and these are crucial to evaluate. Diagnosing this information is critical. The questions asked to assess a patient's VIPs should also be asked of all those in the room with your patient, such as when you are interviewing families or dyads. Their answers often identify each other as their VIPs, thus further strengthening their appreciation for each other. Patients may also reveal as yet undisclosed people or systems that will be crucial in helping them solve their problem. Asking these questions focuses the conversation on who is most important in their life and helps to pinpoint and name these critical relationships. These relationships are often hidden and not spoken about overtly, especially when people are in the depths of their problems. These questions elicit a great deal of information that will be used throughout the conversation, as is exemplified throughout this book. VIPs will be used when negotiating goals as well as when evaluating treatment progress. VIPs may include parents, grandparents, spouses, siblings, teachers, friends, therapists, DCF workers, physicians, community supports, wraparound services staff, employers—

anyone the patient identifies. Table 2–2 lists questions that can be asked to assess a patient's VIPs.

TABLE 2–2.   **Questions that assess a patient's VIPs (very important people)**

- Who are the most important people in your life?
- Who else are the most important people?
- What do you most appreciate about them?
- What else do you appreciate about them?
- How have they been helpful for you?
- How else have they been helpful for you?
- Whose idea was it you come in for treatment?
- Who was worried about you so that they thought coming here would be helpful for you?
- What would tell them that you no longer need to come here for treatment?

Case Illustration: VIP Assessment

Let's continue with Sarah and her mother during their initial treatment encounter.

Anne: Sarah, who are the most important people in your life?
> *Assessing a patient's VIPs is analogous to assessing vital signs such as blood pressure and temperature. VIPs are vital relationships to identify.*

Sarah: My mother.
> *Though many people assume that friends are the VIPs in an adolescent's life, often it is their parents, grandparents, siblings, and other family members.*

Anne: Who else are the most important people in your life?
> *Asking "who else" is a question that digs for more relational resources in a patient's life.*

Sarah: My grandmother, sister, and father.
> *More critical relationships are revealed.*

Anne: Who else is important in your life?
> *I persist in uncovering further relational resources.*

Sarah: My best friend and my boyfriend.

Anne: Who else?

Sarah (*pause*): That's all.
> *This response indicates it is timely to move forward with further questions. I now have a list of her identified VIPs as well as the order in which they were revealed. This gives additional information and can provide clues as to the strengths and difficulties of relationships in her life.*

Anne: What do you most appreciate about your mother?
> *This question is crucial. Often by the time children and parents seek help, they are exhausted, discouraged, and feeling like failures as parents and children.*

For parents to hear their child appreciate things in them is a huge relational deposit. Parents' confidence and competence is greatly increased when they hear directly from their own child how they are appreciated. No compliment is greater for parents than hearing their own child appreciate what they have done for them. I am amazed by how often this causes parents to cry. They have rarely if ever heard these things directly stated, and wow, is it powerful. This simple, yet very powerful question was never directly asked. This question is very healing for the parent and child relationship and creates a strikingly different direction for the conversation. Rather than begin with conflict, pain, and disagreement, early on both the parent and child can agree on their love and appreciation for each other. Positive aspects of their attachment and bond are accentuated. This provides "anesthesia" for the often painful and difficult issues that do come up. The order and choice of questions asked by the therapist are critical. I liken it to being the captain of a ship. It takes gentle and persistent vigilance to keep a ship on course.

SARAH: She has never given up on me.

ANNE: Wow! What else do you appreciate about her?

Asking "what else" digs for more relational strengths.

SARAH: She has never stopped supporting me or judged me. Even with all I have put her through.

ANNE: What else do you appreciate about her?

I persevere in uncovering relationship deposits. These are akin to gold.

SARAH: She is a great mother. She works really hard. I don't know what I would do without her.

ANNE: What else do you appreciate about her?

SARAH: She has a nice fiancé now, and he's been really good to her. He has helped us more than our father has in our whole life.

Notice how the pursuit of "what else" has now uncovered an additional VIP, who as yet had not been identified. Digging for details has paid off.

ANNE: (*I can see mother tearing up, and now direct a question to her based on this response.*) Did you know this about your daughter, how much she appreciates you?

Asking parents directly whether they knew this about their child is very helpful. Although at first glance it may appear obvious, the obvious is often not stated out loud and has tremendous power for both the child and the parent relationship. Parents are often shocked by these responses. Identifying these relational strengths early on builds a parent's competencies while simultaneously identifying and amplifying the child's strengths. And, of course, when mom feels better, kids feel better. These questions are essential in determining not only relational strengths between the parent and child, but also parental strengths. Children know their parents much better than the clinician does, and what the child states are his or her parent's strengths is a much more powerful compliment than what a clinician could say.

MOTHER: No. I never heard her say these things (*crying*).

ANNE: Did you know how important this is to your mom?

This question helps the child appreciate how important she is are in the parent's life, further strengthening their relationship.

SARAH: I just assumed she knew.

ANNE (*asking mom*): Did you know this?

Asking this bidirectionally magnifies their importance to each other.
MOTHER (*still tearful*): I guess I hoped this was the case, but it means a lot to hear it.
ANNE: It is clear how much the two of you care about and love each other.
   I directly compliment their love for one another. It is powerful to state this out loud.
MOTHER: I never heard her say it. It means a lot (*tearful*). I know Bob, my fiancé, has been the first man that has really treated me well. He has really helped me through this and given me the support I need. He really encouraged me to open my eyes and see what was going on and get her the help she needs.
   More positive details of VIPs are revealed.
ANNE: It sounds like Bob is a very important person in your life.
MOTHER: Yes, he is.

At this point, there are many possible directions to go in the conversation. In this case, I chose to continue to ask more about what she appreciates about the other people she identified as important in her life, including her grandmother, sister, father, best friend, and boyfriend. This line of questioning was very valuable and led to a wealth of resources that could easily be left undiscovered if not asked. When asked, Sarah spoke about her grandmother being there for her and about being in debt to her for life. She spoke about her sister as someone whom she cares deeply about and wants to be a better role model for. She spoke about how her best friend was supportive of her treatment and her boyfriend was someone who really understood her. After Sarah's VIPs were identified and amplified, her mother was asked about her VIPs. Assessing VIPs is not only important for the child, but also for parents. Detailing both parent and child VIPs helps to identify and amplify both of their positive relationship attributes, simultaneously building the treatment alliance and, more importantly, the parent and child attachment.

Let's continue to look at this vignette.

ANNE (*asking mother*): Who are the most important people in your life?
MOTHER: My kids. I would do anything for them.
   This is the typical response. For parents, their children are extremely important. This may appear obvious, but to have her mother state this out loud further demonstrates to Sarah how much she is valued.
ANNE: How many children do you have?
   Asking parents about all their children, even those not in the room, helps to further detail their unique social context and elaborate details of their VIPs.
MOTHER: I have two, Sarah and Lisa.
ANNE: How old is Lisa?
MOTHER: She is ten years old.
ANNE: Wow, two beautiful daughters! What do you most appreciate about Sarah?

> *Notice how I have still as yet to ask what their problem is. This will be addressed, but not until a complete assessment of strengths, resources, and VIPs has been identified. Let's digress for a moment and review the basic assumptions in solution-focused therapy. Children want their parents to be proud of them, and parents want their children to succeed and do well in life. Asking parents what they appreciate about their child provides a concrete way for children to hear their parents tell them they are proud of them. Asking children what they are good at and what they appreciate about their parents is a concrete way for parents to hear good things about their child and good things about who they are as a parent. Children and parents both need to and benefit from hearing these things.*

MOTHER: I know she can do anything she puts her mind to. She is smart and very caring when she wants to be.

> *The word "appreciate" often yields more internal strengths.*

ANNE: What else do you appreciate about her?

MOTHER: She is a hard worker and the people at her job love her.

ANNE: Wow. Where did she learn those skills?

> *Asking parents where their children learn skills often results in an indirect compliment to the parent.*

MOTHER: Well, I am a hard worker and don't give up. We've been through a lot together.

ANNE: I can see what a hard worker you are and how you don't give up. Where do you get your strength?

> *A direct and indirect compliment are provided.*

MOTHER: I have faith, and my mother. That really helps.

ANNE (*nodding*): What do you know about Sarah that tells you she will succeed in life?

> *This is an extremely useful question. Even when parents are extremely overwhelmed and feeling hopeless about their children, I have never had a parent not be able to answer this question. It instills hope and reminds both the child and parent about the confidence a parent has in his or her child's potential to succeed in life.*

MOTHER: I know she can succeed in life. She just has to make the right choices and get her head on straight. I've seen her do well in school. She is smart, if she would just put her mind to it.

(*At this point I can also see Sarah appearing more relaxed and positive.*)

This example demonstrates the importance of the ways in which solution-focused interviewing is different from a traditional interview. The questions that are asked and the sequence in which they are asked are unique. Learning solution-focused therapy requires beginning with detailing what people are good at and who are the most important people in their lives.

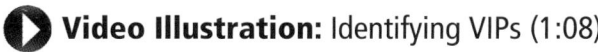 **Video Illustration:** Identifying VIPs (1:08)

Diagnosing and Amplifying Positive Differences (Exceptions)

Positive differences, also known as *exceptions*, are those times when the expected problem could have occurred but did not occur or was less severe (Berg 1994; de Shazer 1988). Positive differences are times when patients are doing things differently than usual and these differences are helpful for them in lessening their problems. Paying attention to these positive differences or exceptions is very important. de Shazer emphasizes that solutions are often built from formerly unrecognized differences (de Shazer 1988). These actions require close attention and meticulous listening on the part of the clinician, as often they go unnoticed by the patient, given how difficult it is to perceive these differences individually (Witkin 2000). For the solution-focused clinician, noticing involves listening with the "third ear" for any possible successes or positive differences that the patient may as yet be unaware of. The act of noticing is difficult to do alone, but through conversation these differences are detected and confirmed with the patient. Noticing positive differences with patients amplifies successes they have already accomplished. Learning solution-focused therapy requires detailed attention and the noticing of positive differences that reveal essential data and resources related to potential solutions for the patient's problems. As Steve de Shazer said: "Where is God? In the space between us" (S. de Shazer, personal communication).

Problem patterns are never rigidly fixed through time and across different situations. There are always times and situations when the problem occurs slightly less frequently or even not at all (de Shazer 1988). Indeed, the fact that a person is aware that there is a problem suggests that he or she is making a comparison to another time or situation when the problem did not exist. For the solution-focused clinician, these exceptions are not to be forgotten, ignored, or considered flukes. Much as a good physician does not want to miss the diagnosis, the solution-focused clinician does not want to miss diagnosing any potential positive differences to problems that may be crucial for successful treatment. These positive differences require the closest attention and signify solutions already occurring within the patient's experience (Nylund and Corsiglia 1994). They bring critical assessment data regarding the details of successes that are indispensable for achievement of the patient's desired goals. Investing the time to amplify these positive differences often yields big returns in terms of positive change. Any time a person does something differently in a positive direction, a change has already occurred and is crucial to scrutinize. Many times patients are unaware that they have done something differently. For the solution-focused clini-

cian, increasing a patient's awareness of these positive differences by noticing them in the conversation amplifies these critical distinctions.

Several useful questions help to diagnose positive differences. These
questions are asked in a specific sequence in order to further magnify these
differences and help people learn the useful patterns they have already
achieved, giving them more confidence that they can do more of these in
the future. Questions asked to identify positive differences are shown in Table 2–3.

TABLE 2–3.   Questions that amplify positive differences (exceptions)

1. Was it different?

2. How was it different?

3. Was it helpful?

4. How was it helpful?

5. How did you do it?

6. How else did you do it?

7. Did others notice a difference?

8. Were things different between you and others when this happened?

The eight questions that are asked in order to diagnose positive differences or exceptions are simple, yet simple does not mean easy. Using these
questions effectively takes fastidious listening and diligence when one is
learning solution-focused therapy. Let's take a closer look at how these
questions amplify a patient's successes. The question "Was it different?"
helps to notice and confirm with patients whether they thought there was
a difference. When a patient says *yes*, agreement is duly noted. Every time
a patient says *yes* to a question and agreement is confirmed with the therapist, engagement and collaboration between the patient and therapist are
strengthened. The next question asked is "How was it different?" This
question reveals several things. Patients usually respond to this question by
talking about times when their problematic behavior was worse. Asking the
question in this way uncovers the symptoms, but instead of highlighting
the problem, it creates a narrative of strength, competence, and hope because the patient has already experienced a triumph. When patients reveal
problematic behaviors in the context of already having accomplished the
overcoming of difficulties, achievements rather than troubles are highlighted and the treatment engagement is enhanced. The symptomatic behaviors are identified, but within a narrative of patient competence.
Solution-focused therapy has been criticized for ignoring the problem and

not giving patients a sense of feeling heard. Asking these questions, in this sequence, addresses some of these concerns. Problematic behaviors are recognized and validated, but they are identified from a narrative in which the patient's strengths are highlighted. The next question asked in this sequence is whether this difference was helpful for them. Asking whether the different behavior is helpful confirms with the patient that this difference was useful for them. This helps patients identify and learn useful behavioral patterns they are already achieving. This reaffirms and validates with patients that they are capable of making changes in their life that are beneficial for them, instilling hope and confidence. This question also creates another opportunity for a *yes* response that promotes the collaborative relationship and strengthens the therapeutic alliance. This query is followed by the question "How was this helpful?" This question elaborates how this difference was valuable for them. This is then succeeded by the question "How did you do it?" This question draws out what they have already done to accomplish the positive difference they accomplished. This question is critical. Behavioral change occurs as a result of actions that a patient does and can do more of so that successes can continue. This is the quintessential concept of solution-focused therapy. When things are working, do more of them, and when things are not working, throw them in the garbage and do something different (de Shazer et al. 2007; Quick 1996).

The identified positive differences can be further amplified by asking patient "how else" they did it. Asking "what else" or "how else" uncovers more details of what patients have accomplished. Asking whether anything was different between them and others when the positive difference occurred highlights how their useful behaviors affect their relationships. Highlighting positive differences between patients and those who are most important in their life has great potential to strengthen the bond and attachments between children and their parents and other VIPs. In this way, positive differences that impact relationships are enhanced. Asking whether others have noticed a difference helps patients see how the differences they made affect those around them. As can be seen from this line of questions, what may seem a small positive difference has tremendous potential to be amplified if it can be noticed and enhanced through these conversational techniques. Every time a positive difference is identified, the same sequence of questioning can be repeated, creating and sustaining a narrative of triumph and achievement for the patient.

Reframing the identified positive differences as skills that a patient already possesses guides the conversation toward competencies versus pathology. Ben Furman has developed a solution-focused approach for children in which problems are transformed into goals by focusing on "kids skills" (Furman 2011). Children as well as adults often dislike being judged abnormal. Instead, both children and adults meet with openness and enthusiasm the challenge of gaining mastery and learning new skills, and they delight in being affirmed as normal, especially by a clinician. Reframing as skills the behavioral actions with which children and parents have already had success reinforces their capabilities to work hard and gain expertise, all of which reinforces their sense of self-efficacy.

Identifying and amplifying positive differences can also be related to diagnostic categories, simultaneously transforming a psychiatric assessment interview into a more positive therapeutic endeavor. For example, paying attention to when children are able to stop and think, focus on their homework, calm down, and manage their frustration provides diagnostic information related to ADHD and mood disorders. (This will be discussed in more detail in Chapter 8, on solution-focused psychiatric assessment.) It is important to amplify positive differences by asking: Was it different? How was it different? Was it helpful? How was it helpful? How did you do it? and so on. Although this sequence of questions may seem mechanistic, patients do not experience it this way. Instead, patients' strengths and competencies are highlighted and useful patterns are recognized, all while simultaneously reinforcing the treatment alliance.

Pausing a conversation to notice positive differences is quite distinct from what most clinicians are taught to do. These positive differences can quickly pass by in a conversation, resulting in lost opportunities and missed positive diagnosis. In the quest for identification of positive differences, there are some potential areas that may be useful to notice and amplify with patients. Table 2–4 lists potential differences to notice with both children and adults. Notice that these positive differences all involve actions. Positive actions are critical to notice. This list is not exhaustive, and your own list will necessarily grow as you learn and become more skilled at solution-focused therapy.

Case Illustration: Diagnosing and Amplifying Positive Differences

Let's continue with the interview with Sarah and her mother. The interview picks up with the conversation about Sarah's mother's relationship with her fiancé and how her mother identified this relationship as helpful for her. Pay attention to how positive differences are identified, conversation is paused, and these differences are amplified.

ANNE: Is this different that you are in a relationship with a man who treats you so well?

Learning solution-focused therapy requires the therapist to put on the conversational brakes whenever there may be an opportunity to identify and amplify a positive difference. Listening in this way is very different from a traditional interview and requires metaphorically growing a "third ear."

TABLE 2–4.   Positive differences to notice with children and adults

Difference in ability to…

- Stop and think
- Make positive, healthy decisions
- Wait and delay gratification
- Say no to negative peer pressure
- Say OK and do what parents ask without arguing
- Cope and manage adversity
- Use words to express their feelings
- Ask for what they need
- Ignore others who are distracting
- Calm down
- Think positively
- Ask for help
- Identify and tolerate uncomfortable feelings
- Get homework done
- Get along better with a parent or sibling
- Do positive things for themselves and others
- Make good decisions
- Focus on work
- Do the right thing
- Manage drug craving
- Cut down on drug use
- Have a sober day
- Attend an AA meeting
- Do something fun with their family
- Do something else instead of harming themselves
- Do something else instead of fighting
- Provide physical affection and comfort to their child
- Play and have fun with their child
- Remain calm when following through on a consequence
- Validate and listen to their child's feelings, including anger, without taking these personally
- Demonstrate appropriate supervision for their child
- Maintain a sense of humor
- Support their child's independence
- Work together as a parental team to help their child with what he or she needs
- Take time to care for themselves
- Appreciate their child's opinions and feelings, even if different from their own

It requires hard work to listen this closely for positive differences, and traditional interviewing techniques have focused on the reverse. In working with parents and children, together or in other dyads, it is important to pause throughout the interview for any potential positive differences.

MOTHER: Yes, very.

Agreement is noted and confirmed.

ANNE: How is this different?

This question amplifies her success while at the same time gathering information that may be helpful.

MOTHER: Before, I was in many difficult relationships where I was not treated well, and unfortunately many of these were seen by my daughter.

This question brings up issues of trauma and domestic violence in a respectful way in which the mother freely reveals the information without being directly asked. Problems are emerging while a narrative of strength and resilience is being built.

ANNE: This must be very difficult for you. Has it been helpful to be in a relationship with a man that treats you well?

I provide emotional validation by tagging the words "for you" at the end of the statement. (This technique will be explained further in the next chapter.) Bridging this "for you" statement to a question that amplifies this difference continues to build the solutions.

MOTHER: Yes, very.

Agreement is noted and confirmed.

ANNE: How has it been helpful?

I continue with the line of questioning to amplify the identified positive difference.

MOTHER: He has supported me with Sarah. He helped me see what a problem she has and really pushed me to get her more help.

More strengths are identified.

ANNE: How else has it been helpful?

This question further elaborates how this difference is helpful for her, gathering more solutions.

MOTHER: I could not have gotten Sarah into treatment without him. He is there for me and for Sarah. She has never had a relationship with a male figure in her life like this.

ANNE: How have you been able to do this, have a relationship with a man who is supportive and helpful for you in your life?

This question is crucial in helping build her self-efficacy and do more of what is working.

MOTHER: I knew I was losing myself and couldn't do it anymore.

ANNE: This must have been very difficult for you. Was this different that you knew you were losing yourself and couldn't do it anymore?

The amplification of positive differences often yields newly undiscovered positive differences that can then be amplified, continuing the solution-building conversation.

MOTHER: Yes.

Agreement is confirmed and noted.

ANNE: How was it different?

Another round of amplification of positive differences is commenced.

MOTHER: It just came to a point where I couldn't stand how my ex-husband was drunk all the time and abusing my children. I just couldn't do it anymore. I had to do it for my children and myself. I had to leave him.

Notice again how problematic behavior is emerging, at her pace, without being directly confronted.

ANNE: That takes tremendous strength and courage to leave. Was it helpful for you to leave him?

A direct compliment is bridged with a question that amplifies this positive difference.

MOTHER: Very.

Agreement noted and confirmed.

ANNE: How was it helpful for you?

The amplification process continues.

MOTHER: The kids. They weren't around all this craziness. There wasn't all the yelling and screaming.

ANNE: How else was it helpful?

MOTHER: I began to realize I could do things without him.

ANNE: Wow! You are an amazingly strong woman. How did you do this?

MOTHER: I couldn't have done it without the support of my sister. She has really supported me in this.

ANNE: How else have you been able to do this?

MOTHER: Before, I wouldn't ask for help and would try to do it all on my own. It just came to a point that I realized I needed more support. I had to ask for help.

ANNE: Was this different for you to ask for help?

Another potential positive difference identified and amplified.

MOTHER: Yes.

ANNE: How was this different?

MOTHER: I would never ask for help or want people to know what was going on. I always thought things would get better, but they never stayed that way.

ANNE: Was it helpful for you to ask for help?

MOTHER: My sister and family have become a lot closer. They have been such great support.

ANNE: It takes a lot of courage to ask for help. How did you do it?

MOTHER: I had to for my children and myself. I couldn't keep going the way it was going. It wasn't working.

As can be seen from this example, pausing the conversation by asking the same line of questions repeatedly reveals more and more strengths and resources, both individually and relationally. Problems came up, but were framed in such a way, through the questions asked, that her skills were amplified and hope increased. The way these questions are asked may seem mechanistic, but rarely do patients notice or seem to care about this. Occasionally I have had an adolescent complain about all the questions I do ask. I remind them of how I warned them of this at the beginning, and that the questions I ask are a tool for me to use in order to help them. Positive differences are also a way to provide compliments to patients. At the end of a session, they can easily be listed to patients, reinforcing their accomplishments, strengthening the treatment alliance, and helping them feel appreciated and validated.

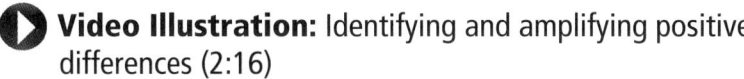 **Video Illustration:** Identifying and amplifying positive differences (2:16)

LEARNING EXERCISE 2: PRACTICING SOLUTION-FOCUSED QUESTIONS

Ask members of a group to break up into groups of three. One person will act as a therapist, one person as a patient, and one person as an observer. Encourage the groups to practice asking each other what they enjoy and are good at, who their VIPs are, and what they most appreciate about them, and then paying attention to positive differences and amplifying them through the line of questioning discussed in this chapter. Have the group switch roles between these exercises. Encourage the observer to pay attention and log all the solution-focused questions asked and how this influenced the direction of the conversation. Have the members talk about what was helpful about this and what they learned through this exercise.

KEY POINTS

- A solution-focused conversation begins with problem-free talk. Problem-free talk is a simple way to build areas of agreement.
- Problem-free talk is not social chit-chat. Skipping problem-free talk puts the clinician at risk of missing crucial resources for the treatment of patients.
- Compliments are important to provide early and frequently throughout a solution-focused conversation.
- Compliments can be either direct or indirect. A good indirect compliment is in the form of a question: "How did you do it?"
- Conversational deposits are important to provide early and can be furnished by asking about areas of enjoyment and talents, as well as by giving compliments.
- Much as a physician is required to obtain vital signs, the solution-focused therapist is required to assess a patient's VIPs.
- For the solution-focused therapist, the notion of a patient is broadened to include the individual patient and his or her VIPs. The VIPs are the social context in which patients must develop their solutions.
- Positive differences, also known as exceptions, are those times when the expected problem could have occurred but did not, or was less severe.
- Positive differences signify solutions already occurring within a patient's experiences, and thus they need to be noticed with the closest attention.

- It is important to amplify positive differences by asking "Was it different?" "How was it different?" "Was it helpful?" "How was it helpful?" and "How did you do it?"

References

Berg IK: Family Based Services: A Solution-Focused Approach. New York, WW Norton, 1994

Berg IK, De Jong P: Engagement through complimenting. Journal of Family Psychotherapy 16:51–56, 2005

Campbell J, Elder J, Gallagher D, et al: Crafting the "tap on the shoulder": a compliment template for solution-focused therapy. Am J Fam Ther 27:35–47, 1999

Cheng MK: New approaches for creating the therapeutic alliance: solution-focused interviewing, motivational interviewing, and the medication interest model. Psychiatr Clin N Am 30:157–166, 2007

De Jong P, Berg IK: Interviewing for Solutions. Belmont, CA, Thomson Brooks/Cole Publishing, 1998

De Jong P, Berg IK: Co-constructing cooperation with mandated clients. Soc Work 46:361–374, 2001

de Shazer S: Clues: Investigating Solutions in Brief Therapy. New York, NY, WW Norton, 1988

de Shazer S, Berg IK, Lipchik E, et al: Brief therapy: focused solution development. Fam Process 25:207–221, 1986

de Shazer S, Dolan Y, Korman H, et al: More Than Miracles: The State of the Art of Solution-Focused Brief Therapy. New York, Haworth, 2007

Furman B: Kids' skills: an innovative and playful way to help children overcome problems. Educating Young Children: Learning and Teaching in the Early Childhood Years 17:24–27, 2011

George E, Iveson C, Ratner H: Briefer: A Solution Focused Manual. London, BRIEF, 2006

Green LS, Oades LG, Grant AM: Cognitive-behavioural solution-focused life coaching: enhancing goal striving, well-being, and hope. The Journal of Positive Psychology 1:142–149, 2006

Kraemer HC, Measelle JR, Ablow JC, et al: A new approach to integrating data from multiple informants in psychiatric assessment and research: mixing and matching contexts and perspectives. Am J Psychiatry 160:1566–1577, 2003

Lambert MJ, Barley DE: Research summary on the therapeutic relationship and psychotherapy outcome. Psychotherapy: Theory, Research, Practice, Training 38:357–361, 2001

Lethem J: Brief solution focused therapy. Child and Adolescent Mental Health 7:189–192, 2002

Nylund D, Corsiglia V: Being solution-focused forced in brief therapy: remembering something important we already knew. Journal of Systemic Therapies 13(1):5–12, 1994

Pichot T, Smock SA: Solution-Focused Substance Abuse Treatment. New York, Routledge/Taylor & Francis Group, 2009

Quick EK: Doing What Works in Brief Therapy: A Strategic Solution Focused Approach. San Diego, CA, Academic Press, 1996

Witkin SL: Noticing. Soc Work 45:101–104, 2000

CHAPTER 3

The Yes-Set

The *yes-set* is a solution-focused skill that involves creating a conversation in which both the clinician and patient say *yes* and agree on as many aspects of the conversation as possible. The yes-set is a metaphor for the patient's acceptance of the intervention message or any therapeutic suggestion (de Shazer 1985; Erickson 2009). Getting the answer *yes* as many times as possible throughout the conversation is another tool that helps build the therapeutic alliance. Developing the yes-set skill involves asking questions that are likely to be answered in the affirmative early on and throughout the interview, and it involves taking the time to pause the conversation in order to confirm these areas of agreement. Yes-set skills also maintain the focus of the conversation on the patient's needs and goals through carefully constructed questions. Constructing a conversation in which enough time is spent talking about areas of agreement strengthens the yes-set. When patients talk about things that they agree on and can say yes to as often as possible, they become less defensive and more eager to engage collaboratively within the conversation.

General Yes-Set Skills

General yes-set skills include verbal and nonverbal responses. Verbal responses include acknowledging a patient's narrative with words such as "yes," "sure," "of course," and "that makes sense." Nonverbal responses include behaviors such as leaning forward, maintaining eye contact, and nodding affirmatively.

The Content Yes-Set

Yes-set areas of agreement include both content and emotions. The *content yes-set* can be defined as the identification and confirmation of elements agreed on within the conversation. These elements begin with strengths and include what the patient identifies as areas of enjoyment, talents, hobbies, very important people in their lives (VIPs), positive differences, coping skills, and identified needs. In contrast to problem areas, it is much easier to agree on what people enjoy, are good at, and appreciate about each other, particularly when you are building engagement simultaneously with multiple people who may have very different goals and perceived views of their problems. In fact, often these problem areas are a bone of contention, and starting off with these issues runs the risk of alienating patients and those most important to them, putting the therapeutic alliance in jeopardy. Initiating the conversation with questions that intensify areas of mutual appreciation and strengths can easily identify domains of agreement among children, parents, and spouses. Children generally are eager to talk about what they are good at, and parents love to hear good things about their child. It helps parents feel they are good parents. These responses make it immediately apparent that all care about and appreciate each other, and (importantly) they are easy to agree on. Building a yes-set accentuates crucial areas of consensus in the dialog, adding conversational "deposits" that build and strengthen relational bonds.

Two questions are particularly helpful in building the content yes-set. These questions were discussed previously (in Chapter 2) in the context of learning how to amplify positive differences. They are:

1. Was this different for you?
2. Was it helpful for you?

Both of these questions confirm with patients that there was a difference and that the difference was helpful for them. In this way, the content of the conversation is verbally agreed on. A greater number of verbal *yes* responses obtained from patients signals that treatment engagement is moving in a positive direction and a collaborative conversation between patient and clinician is mutually strengthening.

 Video Illustration: Building the content yes-set (1:38)

The Emotional Yes-Set

The *emotional yes-set* is defined as the acknowledgment and confirmation of a patient's situation and emotions from the patient's perspective. Noticing emotions and providing validation and empathy is a critical need for all people (Darwin 1896; Lipchik 2002; Plutchik 2000; Rogers 1975). Taking the time to acknowledge and confirm the emotional perspective of patients is another way to build agreement and an important technique in practicing solution-focused therapy (Kiser 1993; Lipchik 2002). In medicine, we are taught that pain is what the patient says it is, and this goes for emotional experiences as well. There is no disagreement about what a patient's feelings are, much as there is no disagreement about what a patient states their level of physical pain is. When a child is feeling angry and disappointed about limits being set, having extra work to do at school, or getting into trouble, it is critical to first take the time to acknowledge how frustrating this must be for him or her. This helps to confirm with the child that you understand and appreciate his or her perspective and goes a long way toward building engagement and the treatment alliance. When parents are feeling angry, exhausted, and overwhelmed with worry about their child, it is paramount to both acknowledge and confirm how difficult this must be for them. There is no argument about feelings. Feelings are what the patients say they are, and are vital to both acknowledge and confirm. Tremendous benefit comes from taking the time to acknowledge and confirm these emotional experiences, and enormous cost results from not doing so. The risk is the patient becoming more defensive, guarded, and distant, derailing the therapeutic alliance. Taking a brief moment to pause the conversation, acknowledge the patient's feelings, and confirm these with him or her helps the therapist stay attuned to the patient's emotional state, further enhancing engagement and collaboration. Much as a good parent stays attuned to the child's needs and emotional states, so too a therapist attempts to remain attuned to the patient's needs and emotional states.

"For You" Linguistic Statements

One language technique that can facilitate the emotional yes-set and provide empathic responses quickly and easily to patients is integrating the words *for you* within statements and questions. These are called *"for you" statements.* Using these words maintains the focus of the conversation linguistically on the patient and his or her needs. "For you" statements can be used in several different ways, and help build agreement within the conversation while providing validation and acknowledgment of the patient's situation and feelings.

The following are examples of "for you" statements used to provide validation for a patient's situation. When an adolescent boy is forced to come in for treatment because his parents are concerned that he was suspended from school, it generally does not help promote conversation or the treatment alliance to ask him why he is here or why he did these things. Instead, the first order of business is to both acknowledge and confirm the experiences from his perspective, for example, saying, *Wow, that must really stink "for you" that you are grounded and can't see your friends*, or saying, *What a bummer "for you" that you have all this extra work and can't play video games*. When an adolescent girl comes to you because her parents are concerned she needs help controlling her anger after she broke several fingers punching a wall, the first thing to acknowledge is how painful this must be "for her" and how it really stinks "for her" that she hurt her hand. Children are frequently surprised by these responses, which are very different from the typical feedback they receive. They are often accustomed to being asked "why" they did this, or told this is "why" they shouldn't have done this. While that all may be relevant, these questions do little to validate their experience, often escalating conflict and disagreement. Reflecting and confirming their feelings with an inquisitive tone and tacking on the words "for you" takes the clinician and parents out of the emotional argument. Confirming the emotional aspects of behaviors from the patient's perspective helps them notice that their current way of doing things is either positively or negatively affecting what they want and need, and can help them move in directions that are more helpful for them. This can enhance their motivation to change and do things differently. There is no arguing that it stinks "for them" that they lost privileges, can't do the things they want, or hurt their hand punching a wall. When children and parents are experiencing conflict, it can help to acknowledge each of their emotional experiences individually, even when they are all in the room together. This often calms all the participants because they are each receiving individual agreement and validation of their unique experiences, allowing the conversation to proceed in a more collaborative manner.

"For you" statements can also be used to acknowledge positive patient experiences, such as what a source of pride it must be "for them" that their child is doing well, or how fantastic it must be "for them" to have accomplished a new skill. Positive "for you" statements reinforce with patients that what they are doing is working for them, and are another way to provide them with indirect compliments.

These "for you" moments of emotional acknowledgment and confirmation must precede a solution-focused question. Otherwise, there is a risk of patients not feeling their experiences are being heard and listened to, thwarting the treatment alliance. Using these words sounds simple, but it can be very difficult to do, especially when parents' or the clinician's own anxiety and frustration is running high. It requires an ability to stay calm and focus on the patient's emotional state rather than reacting to your own anxiety and frustration about being helpful to the patient.

The confirmation received from patients when they say yes or nod affirmatively following "for you" statements indicates that it is then timely to *bridge* these validating responses with a solution-focused question. Pausing the conversation to validate a patient's feelings is often considered mirroring or reflecting, and doing this is also a very important skill in solution-focused therapy (Hersen and Gross 2008; Ivey and Ivey 2007). However, solution-focused therapy moves beyond only mirroring and reflecting by bridging the emotional acknowledgment with a solution-focused question. To omit the solution-focused question would run the risk of keeping a patient in a helpless mode of functioning. To leave out the validation and confirmation of patients' feelings would run the risk of missing critical opportunities to build agreement on their emotional perspective. Both elements are critical when establishing the yes-set.

Integrating "for you" statements within questions is another way to maintain the yes-set and sustain linguistic focus of the conversation on the patient's needs. Table 3–1 lists some examples of how these words are integrated within statements and questions.

TABLE 3–1. **"For you" statements**

Statements that confirm emotional agreement

- That must be so difficult "for you."
- That must be so painful "for you."
- That must be so exhausting "for you."
- That must be so exciting "for you."

Statements integrated within solution-focused questions

- Was that different "for you"?
- How was it different "for you"?
- Was it helpful "for you"?
- How was it helpful "for you"?
- How are "you" able to do this?
- What else was different "for you"?
- What has been better "for you"?
- What else did "you" try to help?

A strong clue that the conversation is not going in a yes-set direction is hearing the comment *Yes, but*… "Yes, but" responses provide strong evidence that something needs to be done differently on the part of the clinician in order to direct the conversation in a more agreeable direction. This is a signal to clinicians that patients need more time having their feelings acknowledged and confirmed and that more attention is needed to asking solution-focused questions that promote agreement.

Case Illustration: The Yes-Set

Karen was a 17-year-old girl who was being treated for opiate dependence in a rehabilitation center. She had suffered three life-threatening overdoses resulting in intensive care treatment. She had been given the choice of going into either a treatment program or adult prison. She decided to choose treatment while awaiting court for two felony convictions. She was externally motivated for treatment by the courts. She was complaining of severe cravings to go out and use. Staff members were frustrated in working with her, complaining of her resistance and lack of motivation for treatment and concerned that she was planning to run off from the program. They were feeling discouraged with her treatment progress and asked the psychiatrist to assess her safety and risk for running away from the program. The following is a portion of the session demonstrating how to develop a yes-set with a challenging adolescent who is externally motivated (mandated) into treatment.

ANNE: What has been better "for you" since you have started this program?
Asking what is better immediately makes an attempt to diagnose positive differences. Especially for patients who are externally motivated, beginning with an exploration for positive differences creates opportunities to highlight achievements and provide compliments, both of which are especially critical to furnish in externally motivated patients.

KAREN: I don't know.
This is a very common response for patients and requires skill to manage. It can mean many things, such as they don't truly know, they don't want to answer, or they don't care if they answer.

ANNE: Hmm (*pause*). I know I ask very difficult questions, and it must be very hard "for you" to be in a program like this. I appreciate that you may need more time to think about this difficult question.
Several things were done to deal with her "I don't know" response. The first was to pause and give her more time. The pause essentially puts the conversational ball back into her court. This was followed first by an emotional yes-set "for you" response validating her experience. Taking responsibility for asking hard questions and appreciating that she may need more time to think about them conveys an appreciation for how difficult these questions are, while communicating your belief in her intelligence (needing more time to "think") about the question.

KAREN: I guess my relationship is better with my family.
These techniques paid off. A positive difference was revealed.

ANNE: Is this different that things are better with you and your family?
The positive difference is amplified through the line of questioning discussed previously in Chapter 2. This builds the content yes-set.

KAREN: Yes.
Agreement is noted and a "yes" response garnered. The more "yes" responses gathered, the stronger the yes-set.

ANNE: How are things better "for you" with your family?

KAREN: I've had a few passes, and I don't feel so annoyed with them. Usually my mother and I just end up fighting all the time and it's miserable (*appearing distressed*).

Another positive difference is uncovered.

ANNE: That must be tough "for you" to feel so annoyed and miserable?

When patients reveal uncomfortable affect, this is a strong indication that they are first in need of a "for you" statement.

KAREN: Yes.

Another yes response was gathered.

ANNE: Was this different "for you" that you felt less annoyed on pass?

After obtaining confirmation that this was difficult for her, I know I can now proceed with further solution-focused questions. I move forward amplifying positive differences discovered.

KAREN: Yes.

She confirmed this difference, collecting another "yes" response.

ANNE: How can you tell this is different, that you are feeling less annoyed?

This question directs her to think and reflect more deeply on this positive difference.

KAREN: I don't know.

ANNE: (*Pause. Smile.*)

She gave another "I don't know" response. It is worth pausing to see if she is willing to answer, given the recent discussion about this response. The smile communicated in a playful way that I am on to her "I don't know" response. It also conveys my comfort with silences, and that I don't personalize or get angry at her responses. It conveys confidence in her ability that she can answer the question with a bit of encouragement.

KAREN: I'm doing more.

The pause paid off, and she did answer the question, identifying another positive difference that can be amplified.

This conversation proceeds by uncovering additional positive differences, including that she finished crocheting a blanket for her family. She acknowledged never finishing anything in her life prior to this, including finishing treatment. Let's look at how the conversation proceeded from this point to illustrate further strategies for building a yes-set with an externally motivated patient.

ANNE: Is it different that you finished something?

KAREN: Yes.

ANNE: How is it different "for you" that you finished this blanket?

KAREN: I usually don't stick things out and have never completed any drug rehab program. I hate being here and think about running every day and going out and using. I've already been here two months. I've never been in a program that long. I hate it and just want to leave.

ANNE: That must be very tough "for you" to stay here and not leave.

The emotional intensity of her previous response indicated she needed a "for you" statement prior to continuing with a solution-focused question.

KAREN: Yes.

ANNE: That's a long time and must be very difficult for you and take a lot of strength to stay here. You could leave. The door is unlocked and other kids have run from this program. Is it different that you have managed to stay in this program for two months?

A direct compliment is bridged with a question, exploring a potential positive difference.

KAREN: Yes. I can't believe I have been here two months.

Another "content yes" response is confirmed.

ANNE: Has it been helpful "for you" to stay?

KAREN: Yes, I guess.

ANNE: How has it been helpful for you?

KAREN: Well, it's better than jail. I don't want leave and end up there.

She has good reason to stay here and a lot to lose if she were to leave. It is much more motivating for her to come to this realization herself. In this way, she realizes it is her choice to determine what would work best for her. This line of questions enhances her internal motivation without directly confronting her.

ANNE: This must be very difficult "for you," to think about the possibility of jail. It sounds like you have thought a lot about this.

Bridging both "for you" statements and compliments with solution-focused questions helps build the yes-set. Taking time to appreciate that she has thought a lot about this respectfully affirms her intelligence and her ability to do what is best for her. This reinforces her skill of thinking things through while validating her ideas about what is in her best interest.

KAREN: Yes. I have thought about it, and I don't want to find out what jail would be like (*appearing distressed*).

ANNE: These must be very difficult and painful things "for you" to think about.

She is appearing emotionally in pain and distressed, a strong clue that more emotional yes-sets are needed prior to asking further questions.

KAREN: I guess. I just get so anxious. I feel like my heart is coming out of my chest.

Notice how more emotional pain is coming forth, including intense anxiety. This is a strong indication that the treatment alliance is strengthening.

ANNE: This must be so difficult "for you." It is extremely tough and takes tremendous skill to be able to know what you are feeling, and tolerate these very uncomfortable feelings without running from the program or going to use drugs. Is this different "for you" that you are able to do this, stay here and cope with these feelings without using?

KAREN: Yes, it is. I just really want to finish something. I only have twenty-nine more days left. I'm more than half way through. It's just one more month (*sounding more hopeful*).

ANNE: How are "you" doing this? Staying here given how difficult these feelings are for you?

KAREN: I just have to go and find something to do. I crochet. I talk with staff and just try to get through the groups.

▶ Video Illustration: Building the emotional yes-set (1:04)

This vignette illustrates how attending to both the emotional and content yes-set guides the conversation toward solutions. The patient feels heard while at the same time solutions are gathered by asking more solution-focused questions. Through this conversation, many successes were identified: her newly discovered mastery of crocheting, her achievement at completing something, a blanket she made for her family, her ability to think about and care how others in her family feel, her appreciation about how her family has stuck with her despite all her difficulties, her ability to think things through so she doesn't end up going to jail, her skill at identifying and coping with painful and uncomfortable feelings without running from the program or using drugs, and her ability to talk with staff. These are all achievements that were identified through these conversational techniques and are critical skills that will help her in her recovery.

LEARNING EXERCISE: PRACTICING "FOR YOU" STATEMENTS

This exercise can be taught to other clinicians and family members, particularly parents who are very frustrated with their children. It is best to have three people involved in this exercise. One person acts as the therapist, one as the patient, and one as an observer. Have the patient complain about something that is troubling him or her for 2 minutes. Then ask the therapist to bridge "for you" responses or compliments prior to asking solution-focused questions. Then ask the observer, patient, and therapist to talk about what this experience was like for them. This simple exercise helps to teach how "for you" statements and compliments can help maintain a solution-focused conversation.

KEY POINTS

- Constructing a conversation in which enough time is spent talking about areas of agreement strengthens the yes-set.

- General yes-set skills involve verbal and nonverbal skills such as saying "yes, of course," leaning forward, and nodding affirmatively.

- The *content yes-set* consists of identified areas of agreement, including areas of enjoyment, talents, and positive differences.

- Asking patients whether potential positive differences are different for them or helpful for them helps to garner *yes* responses. The more *yes* responses, the better.

- When a clinician hears the patient say "yes, but," this is a strong indication something needs to be done differently on the part of the clinician.

- The *emotional yes-set* is the acknowledgment and confirmation of patients' situation and emotions from their perspective.

- Tacking on the words "for you" can help build the emotional yes-set.

- Bridging "for you" statements and compliments prior to asking a solution-focused question helps to build the yes-set and build the therapeutic alliance.

- In working with externally motivated patients, it is critical to provide enough compliments and "for you" statements prior to moving forward with solution-focused questions.

References

Darwin C: The Expression of the Emotions in Man and Animals. New York, D. Appleton, 1896

de Shazer S: Keys to Solution in Brief Therapy. New York, WW Norton, 1985

Erickson MH: Further clinical techniques of hypnosis: utilization techniques. 1959. Am J Clin Hypn 51:341–362, 2009

Hersen M, Gross AM: Handbook of Clinical Psychology, Vol 2: Children and Adolescents, New York, Wiley, 2008

Ivey AE, Ivey MB: Essentials of Intentional Interviewing: Counseling in a Multicultural Society. Belmont, CA, Thomson Brooks/Cole, 2007

Kiser DJ: The integration of emotion in solution-focused therapy. Journal of Marital and Family Therapy 19:235–244, 1993

Lipchik E: Beyond Technique in Solution-Focused Therapy: Working With Emotions and the Therapeutic Relationship. New York, Guilford, 2002

Plutchik R: Emotions in the Practice of Psychotherapy: Clinical Implications of Affect Theories. Washington, DC, American Psychological Association Press, 2000

Rogers CR: Empathic: an unappreciated way of being. The Counseling Psychologist 5:2–10, 1975

CHAPTER 4

Language Skills in Solution-Focused Therapy

A therapeutic conversation is no more than a slowly evolving and detailed, concrete, individual life story stimulated by the therapist's position of not-knowing and the therapist's curiosity to learn. It is this curiosity and not-knowing that opens conversational space and thus increases the potential for the narrative development of new agency and personal freedom.

—Harlene Anderson and Harold A. Goolishian

Attention to Language

Paying attention to how questions are constructed, incorporating the patient's language and exact words, and using suppositional words are all essential skills to acquire in learning to speak the solution-focused therapy language. Language is an essential ingredient in any form of communication. Human systems are language meaning-generating systems (Anderson and Goolishian 1988). Every person has his or her own unique way of using words, talking, and communicating. In essence, we each have our own personal dialect. Common to all forms of therapy is the observation that the therapist and the patient are having a conversation—using language (de Shazer and Berg 1992). In solution-focused therapy, this requires speaking the dialect of the patients with whom we converse—quite a daunting task at first glance, but possible when you learn the skills needed to accomplish this undertaking. All the questions asked by a solution-focused therapist are designed to elicit the patient's view of the problem and of the solution (Berg and de Shazer 1993), and this requires understanding and exploring what patients mean by the words and phrases they speak. It demands paying attention to idiosyncratic ways in which they use certain words, repeating their exact words within the formulation of questions and responses, and exploring what they mean by the particular words they speak. Meaning becomes a function of the relationship, and understanding is always a matter of negotiation between the participants. As Anderson and Goolishian state, "Meaning and understanding are developed by individuals in conversation with each other in their attempts to understand other persons and things, others' words and action" (Anderson and Goolishian 1988).

In solution-focused therapy the clinician enters the relationship and the conversation as a learner, with the patient's meaning taking precedence over the language and meanings of the therapist (Anderson and Goolishian 1992). This demands intense concentration and listening. When a patient hears a clinician use the patient's exact words and take the time to understand what they mean in detail, this promotes engagement and a collaborative working relationship (Anderson 2012). The careful and detailed attention to using a patient's exact words is analogous to a surgeon's deliberate use of a scalpel. Just as a surgeon is very skilled when maneuvering a scalpel, a clinician is meticulous when speaking, rigorously and conscientiously using the exact words of patients.

Vague words are particularly important to clarify with patients. Patients often talk about wanting to be happy, have more self-esteem, feel less stressed, be more open about things, have their children behave, have more self-respect, not get so upset, live a more balanced life, and feel more confident. These words mean different things to different people and are important to define with them. For example, patients may say they want to improve their self-esteem. *Self-esteem* is a rather vague word and can mean different things to different people depending on their unique personal dialect. As Table 4–1 shows, this one word can be integrated within a variety of solution-focused questions to demonstrate how to begin to speak and understand a patient's dialect.

Integrating the patient's exact words into solution-focused questions conveys respect by demonstrating how attentively the clinician is listening. This mode of listening requires carefully scrutinizing every word that a patient speaks. All questions the clinician asks are formulated from the patient's last response or an earlier answer (De Jong and Berg 1998). Solution-focused therapy is not geared toward forcing positives into a problem-saturated story. It requires great skill in constructing useful solution-focused questions that incorporate and echo a patient's key words while consulting with them on the meaning of key words they speak. The following case illustrates how to construct solution-focused questions incorporating a patient's language. Shared

---

**TABLE 4–1.   Example of integrating a patient's language into solu-
tion-focused questions**

- What do you mean by "self-esteem"?
- Suppose you had all the self-esteem you need, what would you be doing differently?
- What else would you be doing differently when you had all the self-esteem you need?
- What would others important in your life notice you doing differently when your self-esteem has improved?
- On a scale of 1–10, where 10 is you are satisfied with the amount of self-esteem you have and 1 is the opposite, where would you rate it now?
- What makes the number not lower?
- What else makes the number not lower?
- What would make the number one point higher?
- Where do you think your VIPs [very important people] would rate your self-esteem from 1–10 supposing they were in the room with us?
- What would be different between you and others who are most important in your life when your self-esteem improves?

---

words that the patient and clinician both speak are highlighted to illustrate how a shared dialect is constructed.

Case Illustration: Using a Patient's Language in Conversation

Destiny was a 16-year-old girl who was receiving treatment for anxiety, depression, and addiction. Her mother suffered from trauma and depression and had difficulties caring for her throughout her life. As a result, Destiny was placed in the custody of her maternal grandmother. Destiny had remarkable strengths, as demonstrated by her decision to turn herself in after being on the run from her family for over 2 months. She came into treatment voluntarily with the goals of getting sober and improving her relationships with her family.

ANNE: What's been better since I last saw you?
   The session begins by asking what is better, immediately exploring for positive differences.
DESTINY: I'm leaving soon, just a few weeks away.
ANNE: Wow, that's great! You have worked very hard here. What else is better?
   A direct compliment precedes digging for more details of success.
DESTINY: My mother is working on getting custody back for me. She is saving money for an apartment.
   An important positive difference is disclosed and will be amplified.
ANNE: Is that different for your mother?
DESTINY: Yes. She's never done this before.

ANNE: Has it been helpful for you?

DESTINY: Yes.

ANNE: How has it been helpful?

DESTINY: I don't want to make myself seem like the cause of this, but I think because I am doing good things for myself, she is trying harder to do things for me.

ANNE: Of course, that makes sense. What good things do you think she sees you doing for yourself?

Notice how I choose to highlight the positive words she speaks within a solution-focused question.

DESTINY: I'm not running from this program.

ANNE: What else does she see you doing that is good for yourself?

More details of positive actions she is taking are amplified.

DESTINY: I'm not asking to leave this program early, and we are communicating a lot better.

ANNE: What do you mean communicating better?

The meanings of vague words are explored in detail.

DESTINY: I know how to keep conversations smoother. I have learned to let things go.

ANNE: What do you mean let things go?

Asking patients what they mean by the words they speak facilitates a shared dialect. Notice how positive words were highlighted.

DESTINY: If something is bothering me about my mom, I just quit talking about it.

ANNE: Is that different for you, how you are able to quit talking about it?

I incorporate the word "able" within the amplification of positive difference query, gently suggesting the patient is "able."

DESTINY: Yes, very!

ANNE: How is it different?

DESTINY: I know the discussion will not go anywhere and it's not the right time.

ANNE: Has this been helpful for you?

DESTINY: Yes.

ANNE: How has it been helpful for you?

DESTINY: I just want to end the phone call on a good note.

ANNE: What do you mean "good note"?

DESTINY: I want our relationship to be more positive.

ANNE: These are impressive skills. How have you been able to develop these communication skills so you end the phone calls on a good note?

A direct and an indirect compliment are furnished incorporating her language.

DESTINY: I just don't let things get to me. I take deep breaths and think about things first.

ANNE: What do you mean "think about things"?

More of her positive language is explored.

DESTINY: I think how it's really not going to change my life to keep arguing with her, and nobody gets what they want from the conversation.

ANNE: Wow! I am impressed how you are able to think things through like this. What do you think you need from conversations with your mother instead of arguing?

DESTINY: I need to be able to get my point across in a calm manner and not demand things.

ANNE: I am impressed with how you have thought about this. What do you mean "get your point across"?

DESTINY: I used to want, want, want! This urgent want, to get what I want and screw you if I don't. Now I am asking for things.
Another positive difference has been identified.

ANNE: Is that different how you are able to ask for things?

DESTINY: Yes.

ANNE: How is it different for you to ask for things?

DESTINY: I used to give her so much attitude and the "F— -its." I would be rude and not care.

ANNE: Has it been helpful for you to ask for things?

DESTINY: Yes.

ANNE: How has it been helpful?

DESTINY: We are getting along better and getting closer. She is beginning to trust me more.

ANNE: How have you been able to do this, ask for things instead of demanding things?

DESTINY: I say "anyway."

ANNE: What do you mean "anyway"?

DESTINY: When the conversation is going in a bad direction, I say "anyway" and change the subject to something more neutral. I don't try to manipulate the conversation to get what I want.

ANNE: What do you do instead of manipulating the conversation?

DESTINY: I don't try and bend the rules. I say OK.

ANNE: "OK" is a beautiful word. Parents love that word. Did you know that?

DESTINY (*smiling*): I never really thought about that.

ANNE: What else do you do instead of manipulating the conversation?
I detail what else she would "do instead," maintaining the positive direction of the conversation.

DESTINY: I leave it as it is. Before, I would keep talking and keep bringing it up again and again to badger her until she gave in.

ANNE: What do you mean by leave it as it is?

DESTINY: I listen and just let it go. I don't keep badgering her.

This case illustrates how meticulous attention to using a patient's language within solution-focused questions can uncover many strengths and useful patterns that could easily be missed. Using a patient's words within the conversation strengthens the collaborative relationship, building a shared solution-focused dialect between the patient and the clinician.

The Nonassuming Stance

The nonassuming stance is another important linguistic skill to master when learning solution-focused therapy. This stance was influenced by the work of Anderson and Goolishian (Anderson and Goolishian 1988, 1992).

The nonassuming position entails a general attitude in which the therapist's actions communicate an abundant, genuine curiosity, a need to know more about what has been said, rather than preconceived opinions and expectations about the patient, the problem, or what must be changed (Anderson and Goolishian 1992). It means putting patients into the position of being the experts on their own lives and having faith that they have the resources and skills necessary to solve their problems. This can be especially challenging for physicians given the culture of training that emphasizes the physician as an expert in problem detection and pathology-based diagnosis. In solution-focused therapy, clinicians are not limited by their own theoretical knowledge of diagnosis, disease, and treatments, but instead use their expertise in asking questions with the goal of needing to learn more of what was just said from the patient.

Learning how to put aside one's own preconceived assumptions and frame of reference can be a formidable challenge. The nonassuming stance requires clinicians to maintain a genuine curious demeanor when talking with patients, guiding the conversation with solution-focused questions rather than statements and interpretations. This stance conveys a wish and a need to know more, especially when positive differences, exceptions, and strengths are identified (Anderson and Goolishian 1992). Clinicians put themselves in the position of being informed by the patient through the use of meticulously formulated questions. This requires clinicians to suspend their own frame of reference and listen to the patient's story and exact words from his or her unique perspective (De Jong and Berg 2002). The ability to maintain a nonassuming stance requires methodically, and at times painstakingly, asking well-constructed questions incorporating a patient's exact language. The act of asking questions conveys a working belief that patients have the answers to solve their problems. Incorporating their language within the questions facilitates this stance.

Maintaining this stance does not mean ignoring our training or expertise. It also does not mean ignoring child protective, legal, and safety concerns. It does, however, require having faith and proceeding in the belief that patients have the resources and strengths, once these are discovered and diagnosed, to solve problems in their own unique way. The solution-focused clinician is the expert on the therapeutic process. The patient is the expert on his or her life. This conveys a profound respect for the human dignity of each of our patients.

It can be very difficult to set aside our own preexisting assumptions regarding our patients. Hearing patients' stories from their frame of reference without filtering the conversation through our own beliefs and experiences can be a very arduous task and takes considerable skill and awareness, especially in emotionally charged situations where patients are doing potentially harmful things to themselves or others. These situations create the normative reaction of wanting to help, give advice, and fix things for the patient. In these circumstances, it can be particularly challenging to manage one's own anxiety, suspend one's own frame of reference, and hear the story from the patient's point of view. Two questions are especially useful in situations in which patients are engaging in harmful behaviors. The first is the "good reason" question (de Shazer and Berg 1986). The second is the "how is this helpful" question. The basic format is as follows:

1. You must have a good reason for _____ [fill in the blank with the harmful actions].
2. How is this helpful for you? (referring to harmful actions)

Harmful behaviors may include drug use, suicidal thoughts, self-harming behaviors, abusive behaviors to others, staying in a domestically violent relationship, and having unprotected sex, to name a few. Behaviors such as these often cause a clinician understandable anxiety. Remaining calm and managing your own anxiety is the first challenge. Having questions that you can pull out of your back pocket during these situations goes a long way toward helping you remain unflustered and in control of the therapeutic process. Asking patients what their "good reasons" are for their behaviors and asking "how these behaviors are helpful for them" conveys to patients that they are engaging in these behaviors because in some way they are useful and beneficial for them. Beginning the line of questions by asking patients how harmful behaviors are helpful often eventually leads the conversation to the point of asking, but in a nonconfrontational tone, how these behaviors are *un*helpful for them, while also conveying your faith and belief that, unless the contrary is proven, they are choosing these behaviors because they are in some way useful for them. These questions also magnify ambivalence in a positive and respectful way.

The following vignette illustrates the nonassuming stance. Notice in this example that nearly every response is a solution-focused question that was formulated from the patient's prior response, incorporating her words. This technique maintains the patient in the role of the expert on her solutions, while the clinician is the expert at guiding the conversation. This process of questioning is what sustains the nonassuming stance.

Case Illustration: The Nonassuming Stance

Maria was a 16-year-old girl who was referred for treatment of drug addiction at a residential treatment center for substance dependence. She was externally motivated (mandated) into treatment after failing multiple drug tests and being charged with several accounts of assault and battery. She had been living with her 82-year-old maternal great-grandmother for the past three years after being kicked out of her mother's house. There was a restraining order against her biological father because of his assaultive actions and his status as a registered sex offender. Maria had been hospitalized several times for detoxification from drugs and for suicidal and self-harming behaviors. The staff was concerned about mood swings, irritability, defiance, and regressive behaviors. They were also concerned about her future, given that her grandmother had stated she could no longer care for her and keep her safe in her home. The following is an excerpt from the initial conversation with Maria.

ANNE: Hi, Maria. Thank you for coming in to talk with me today. Would it be OK for me to ask you a few questions and see how I could be most helpful to you? Some of these questions can be quite difficult. I will try my best to be helpful for you.

MARIA: OK.

ANNE (*I notice she is wearing many hand-made bracelets on her wrist.*): Wow, those are nice bracelets you are wearing.

MARIA: I made them myself.

A skill has been revealed and is important to amplify.

ANNE: Wow, all of them? How many are there?

Detailing this skill conveys my interest in her achievements.

MARIA (*counting them*): Sixteen.

ANNE: They are all beautiful, yet unique. Did you design them yourself?

I respond with a direct and indirect compliment.

MARIA: Yes. I learned how to make them here.

ANNE: How did you learn to make them?

Asking how she learned to make the bracelets communicates an openness to learn more about her skill, putting her in the role of accomplished bracelet maker. While asking about her bracelets may at first appear unrelated to the problems at hand, it is critical in conveying belief in her capabilities and talents.

MARIA: I learned from other girls and the staff. I am also learning how to crochet. I started making a blanket for my two-year-old niece.

Her response uncovered several strengths, which can then be amplified.

ANNE: Wow! You are learning a lot of new things. Is this different for you?

I decide to inquire whether her openness in learning new skills is a positive difference.

MARIA: I guess so. I'm not spending all my time getting and using drugs.

Confirmation is obtained, and another positive difference is revealed.

ANNE: What are you doing instead of spending all your time getting and using drugs?

When patients answer questions in the negative (i.e., not spending time getting and using drugs), it is very useful to ask what they are doing instead. The question does not assume I know what she is doing as an alternative. It conveys a curiosity to know the more positive behaviors she was engaging in lieu of spending time getting and using drugs.

MARIA: I'm forced to be here. There's nothing much to do here, so I've had more time to think about things.

She reveals another potential positive difference.

ANNE: It must be difficult for you to be forced to be here. Is this different that you are thinking more about things?

I pair an emotional yes-set response "for you" with a positive difference question.

MARIA: Yes.

ANNE: How is this different for you?

The amplification of positive difference questions continues. Every one of her responses is followed with a carefully constructed question that conveys my desire to learn more from her, setting aside my own assumptions and preconceived ideas.

MARIA: I used to spend all my time getting and using drugs. I wouldn't have time to think about anything else.

Her problems are being revealed, but from a narrative of her strength.

ANNE: How else is it different that you are thinking things through more?

MARIA: I used to not care about anyone. It was all about me getting my drug.

ANNE: I am impressed by how hard you are working thinking about things. Has it been helpful for you to think more about things?

Another compliment is paired with a solution-focused question.

MARIA: I guess so.

ANNE: How has it been helpful for you to think more about things?

MARIA: I realize how important my family is for me. My sister won't even let me talk to my niece. She doesn't trust me (*appearing in more distress*).

She begins to talk more about the VIPs in her life and discloses further problems.

ANNE: That must be very difficult for you, to not be able to talk with your niece.

I provide an emotional yes-set response incorporating her experience.

MARIA: Nodding.

ANNE: There must be a "good reason" for your sister not letting you see her?

Asking the "good reason" question conveys a nonjudgmental stance and demonstrates a genuine curiosity to understand her perspective.

MARIA: She won't let any of us see her. Ever since DCF came and talked to me and then they went to talk to her, she won't let any of us see her family.

People are more likely to reveal sensitive information when they believe you are on their side and genuinely listening to them without judgment or assumptions.

ANNE: It sounds like it has been very difficult for you and your family. How have you been coping with this?

MARIA: I just am trying hard here to get sober again. I was sober for six months in the past, and want to get back on track.

She discloses positive goals and reveals additional strengths after asking how she has been coping.

ANNE: Is that different for you that you want to get sober again and get back on track?

As can be seen from these illustrations, the clinician is the expert on the therapeutic process; however, the patient is the expert on his or her life.

Because of the way the clinician responded, incorporating the patient's own key words within solution-focused questions, a shared dialect was co-constructed between clinician and patient with new meanings and possibilities generated. The role of the therapist is that of a conversational artist whose expertise is in the area of creating space for new, different, and useful conversations for the patient (Anderson and Goolishian 1988).

 Video Illustration: Attention to language (1:10)

Bridging Statements That Promote Solution Building

Bridging statements are types of conversational responses that can help to maintain a conversation directed toward solution building. These responses are helpful with all patients, but particularly when patients are in distress, very problem-focused, and externally motivated. Bridging statements include the use of general, emotional, and content yes-set responses as described in Chapter 3; compliments as described in Chapter 2; and meticulous attention to and use of a patient's language, particularly positive words as described in this chapter. Pairing bridging statements with solution-focused questions assists the clinician in co-constructing a strength-based narrative with patients.

 Video Illustration: Bridging statements (1:37)

LEARNING EXERCISE IN PAYING ATTENTION TO LANGUAGE:
THE THREE-HEADED THERAPIST

If possible, break into groups of at least five, but no more than six, in which one person takes the role of patient and two or more people act as therapists. It is also helpful, if possible, to have one person act as an observer of the group, refereeing to ensure that the structure of the exercise is maintained. Have the patient talk about a problem and then have the therapists take turns responding with *only* one statement that is based *only* on what the patient spoke about immediately before. After each patient response, a different "head" of the therapist responds, practicing using solution-focused bridging statements. The group can also practice using any of the questions discussed previously from the prior chapters. Have the observer record the number of compliments, solution-focused questions, uses of a patient's exact words, yes-set responses, and "for you" responses that each therapist used, and discuss with the group. After 3–4 minutes, stop and explore what it was like for each of the participants. In particular, ask the acting patient to reflect on what were the most helpful questions or responses for him or her. For those acting as therapists, was it more difficult than imagined? Did the conversation slow down? Was it difficult to maintain a nonassuming stance putting one's own assumptions on hold? You can then have the group switch roles to experience this exercise from differing perspectives.

KEY POINTS

- Creating a shared dialect with patients requires meticulously paying attention to key words patients use, incorporating these words within solution-focused questions, and exploring what is meant by particular words spoken.

- Meaning and understanding are developed in conversation between clinician and patient.

- In solution-focused therapy, the clinician enters the relationship as learner, with the patient's meaning taking precedence over the language and meaning of the therapist.

- Highlighting the positive words a patient speaks helps build a solution-focused conversation.

- The act of questioning conveys that patients have the resources to solve their own problems.

- A solution-focused clinician guides the conversation with questions rather than interpretations.

- The solution-focused clinician is the expert on the therapeutic process. The patient is the expert on his or her life.

- The nonassuming stance requires the clinician to maintain a genuine curious demeanor and a need to know more, especially when positive differences and strengths are identified.

- When patients are engaging in harmful behaviors, asking them their "good reason" or "how their behavior is helpful" maintains the nonassuming stance while simultaneously amplifying ambivalence in a nonjudgmental way.

References

Anderson H: Collaborative relationships and dialogic conversations: ideas for a relationally responsive practice. Fam Process 51:8–24, 2012

Anderson H, Goolishian HA: Human systems as linguistic systems: preliminary and evolving ideas about the implications for clinical theory. Fam Process 27:371–393, 1988

Anderson H, Goolishian H: The client is the expert: a not-knowing approach to therapy, in Social Construction and the Therapeutic Process. Newbury Park, CA, Sage, 1992, p 25

Berg IK, de Shazer S: Making Numbers Talk: Language in Therapy, in The New Language of Change: Constructive Collaboration in Psychotherapy. Edited by Friedman S. New York, Guilford, 1993, pp 5–24

De Jong P, Berg IK: Interviewing for Solutions. Belmont, CA, Thomson Brooks/Cole Publishing, 1998

De Jong P, Berg IK: Interviewing for Solutions. Pacific Grove, CA, Brooks/Cole, 2002

de Shazer S, Berg IK: Doing therapy: a post-structural re-vision. Journal of Marital and Family Therapy 18:71–81, 1992

de Shazer S, Berg IK, Lipchik E, et al: Brief therapy: focused solution development. Fam Process 25:207–221, 1986

CHAPTER 5

Scaling Questions and the Miracle Question

There is magic in numbers.
—Steve de Shazer

Scaling questions ask patients to rate their priorities, goals, satisfaction, problems, coping strategies, successes, motivation for change, safety, confidence, treatment progress, and hope on a numerical scale from 1–10. These questions have great versatility and can be used to assess the patient's perception of almost anything (Berg 1994). They are an essential solution-focused tool that helps to measure myriad patient issues, and they can be asked from a multitude of perspectives. They are quick, simple, and easy to ask, making them especially useful for busy clinicians struggling with increasing workloads and briefer appointment times. Scaling questions can be adapted in endless ways. Solution-focused scales are self-anchored rather than normed scales. The patient, not the doctor, defines what a 3 or 7 or 10 means. Scaling questions are used to facilitate treatment and are based on patients' perceptions (Berg and de Shazer 1993). Patients more readily take ownership of their treatment goals and progress when asked to rate them on a scale. Scaling questions help direct the treatment toward what patients want and what is most important to them, increasing their motivation and confidence to change and helping to facilitate agreement among patient, clinician, and others participating in treatment (Berg and de Shazer 1993). Scaling questions can also help defuse intense emotion in a conversation. Scaling questions are often much less conflict ridden than other types of questions. Numbers are numbers. Scaling questions can dramatically lessen the affective tone of emotionally charged issues.

Solution-focused scaling questions are constructed in such a way that the number 10 highlights a positive aspect, such as satisfaction, the problem being solved, progress in treatment, or confidence in ability. They are not negatively constructed as is often the case with scaling questions used in other treatment modalities, such as how much worry, anger, or pain a number 10 connotes. This is an important point. Scaling questions are not used to measure the extent of the problem, but rather the scope of the solution. For example, rather than measuring how angry a child is from 1–10, a solution-focused scale would measure how well a child is able to calm down, from 1–10, where 10 is being satisfied with their ability to calm down and 1 is the opposite. Table 5–1 lists potential scaling questions.

Scaling questions are not unique to this therapy. Pain scales are routinely used in medicine to gauge how much medication is needed for patients. They are simple to use, and responding does not require sophisticated intellectual ability. Scaling questions afford patients a simple way to communicate emotional and cognitive states, measure confidence toward attaining goals, and evaluate safety and coping ability. Scaling questions are also helpful in generating small next steps and evaluating where patients are in relation to their goals of treatment. They can be used to determine when patients are ready to end treatment. Asking patients what number, from 1–10, would tell them they no longer need to be in treatment collaboratively evaluates their treatment progress.

Scaling questions can metaphorically bring the patient's VIPs (very important people) rapidly into the office. Asking children to tell you how they think their mother, father, teacher, or siblings would rate their ability to calm down, get their work done, or get along from 1–10 quickly brings perspectives of others into the conversation. Let's recall how problems are solved (as discussed in Chapter 1). Either the problem goes away, or the patient and the patient's VIPs no longer view the issues at hand as problematic. For this reason, assessing whether the problem is solved from the perspective of both the patient and the VIPs is critical.

Scaling questions are of great value in working with externally motivated (mandated) patients. For example, when an adolescent experiences using drugs as very helpful, sees no problems with the behavior, and appears resistant to treatment, asking him or her to rate how helpful drugs are from 1–10 (where 10 is they are very helpful and 1 is the opposite) from the perspective of parents, teachers, probation officer, or other VIPs in his or her life can help amplify ambivalence. Amplifying ambivalence in an externally motivated patient is the first order of business. Scaling questions can greatly assist with this task. This gets back to how critical it is to know who

TABLE 5–1.	Potential scaling questions

- On a scale of 1–10, supposing that 10 is you are satisfied that your problem is solved and 1 is the opposite, where would you rate things now?
- What makes the number not lower?
- What else makes it not lower?
- What would it take to raise it by one point?
- What else would make it one point higher?
- On a scale of 1–10, where 10 is fully confident and 1 is the opposite, how confident are you that you can achieve your goals?
- Suppose I were to ask your VIPs how confident they are of your ability to achieve your goals from 1–10, where 10 is they are fully confident and 1 is the opposite, where do suppose they would rate you?
- What makes it not lower?
- What would make it one point higher?
- On a scale of 1–10, where 10 is you know you have what it takes to achieve your goals and 1 is the opposite, what number would you give?
- On a scale of 1–10, where 10 is the day after the miracle and 1 is the opposite, where would you say things are now? [See next section for discussion of miracle question]
- What makes it not lower?
- What would make it one point higher?
- On a scale of 1–10, where 10 is you are confident you can stay safe and 1 is the opposite, where would you say you are?
- On a scale of 1–10, where 10 is you are coping and managing despite all the obstacles and challenges and 1 is the opposite, where would you rate yourself?
- On a scale of 1–10, where 10 is you have many reasons for living and 1 is the opposite, where would you say you are now?
- What makes it not lower?
- What would make it one point higher?
- Suppose I were to ask your VIPs how confident they are that you will stay safe from 1–10, where 10 is they are sure you can keep yourself safe and 1 is the opposite, where would they rate you?
- Suppose 10 is the behavior you are doing is the most helpful you can imagine and 1 is the opposite, where would you rate how helpful your behavior is?
- Suppose I were to ask your VIPs how helpful they think these behaviors are from 1–10, with 10 being the most helpful and 1 being the opposite, where would they rate them?

the VIPs are in every patient's life. Many patients, especially children and adolescents, find it easier to answer scaling questions from the perspectives of those most important in their lives.

Scaling questions can be used to help parents, children, spouses, other family members, and treatment providers understand each other's perspectives. When parents and children are asked to rate each other's perspectives, they gain knowledge about each other's point of view. All parties become more attentive and interested. John Lutz has developed a playful way to incorporate scaling questions with families. He calls it the *prediction game*. He asks children to predict how their parents would rate them, and he asks parents to predict how their children would rate them. The game is fun for both parents and children and helps them gain understanding of each other's perspectives and needs in a nonconfrontational way (J. Lutz, personal communication).

Scaling questions can quickly assess the health of relationships in a patient's life. The strength of a patient's VIP relationships is critical to assess. Much as it is important for a physician to assess blood pressure, weight, and laboratory values, it is imperative to assess the health of a patient's relationships. Asking how things are "between" patients and their VIPs from 1–10 rapidly assesses the strength and health of their relationship. Asking what makes the number not lower amplifies positive qualities of their relationships. Asking what else makes it not lower uncovers further positive qualities of relationships. Asking what it would take to raise it by one point helps patients think about small, doable next steps to improve their relationships.

Scaling questions can also be used to assess coping abilities. Asking a mother how she is coping with her child's difficulties, on a scale of 1–10, provides empathy while directing the conversation toward what she is doing to cope and what she needs to do to increase this skill. When parents bring their children in for treatment, they are rarely asked how they are coping and managing. When asked this, parents often become tearful. No one has asked them. Asking how they are coping conveys deep appreciation for what they are doing, while also gathering crucial information. Plenty of research demonstrates that treating maternal depression has a large positive effect size in the treatment of children (Pilowsky et al. 2008; Weissman et al. 2006; Wickramaratne et al. 2011). Asking parents how well they are managing to stay calm from 1–10 assesses this skill in a nonjudgmental way, while directing the conversation to ways they are staying calm and then to the next small steps to gain mastery in this area.

Scaling questions can also be used to amplify strengths, positive differences, and successes. Asking patients how confident they are, from 1–10, that they can continue doing the things that are helping them is just the first step toward magnifying a patient's success. After a patient gives a number, it is then important to question what makes the number NOT lower. This enables more successes to be uncovered and amplified, increasing a patient's hope and confidence by highlighting what he or she has already accomplished. Only after this is investigated is it time to examine what it would take to raise the number by one point—not all the way to a 10, just one small step. This helps patients formulate realistic small next steps toward achieving their goals. One of the biggest goals of a solution-focused therapist is to help patients stay focused on moving forward toward their goals. Scaling questions are fundamental to accomplishing this objective.

As with other solution-focused questions, it is important to amplify details of successes and goals. A very useful question to amplify successes is the "What else" question. What else makes the number not lower? What else? This affords opportunities to compliment patients on successes they have already accomplished, giving them hope in their ability to move forward toward their goals. What would it take to raise it by one point? What else? What else? Learning solution-focused therapy is like digging for gold. Successful prospectors do not stop in their pursuit of wealth. Solution-focused therapists do not stop in their pursuit of strengths and resources.

When patients give a low number, it is still possible to maintain a solution-focused conversation. The first order of business is to validate how difficult this situation is "for them," providing an emotional yes-set response. This can then be followed by coping questions. Even if patients give a low number, such as 2 or 3, it is still critical to ask what makes the number not lower than that. Asking patients where they get their strength to continue on, despite all their difficulties and problems, is a form of indirect compliment that encourages them to appreciate their own strength and resilience.

Having an erasable whiteboard and a basket of markers in your office can be of great assistance when you ask scaling questions. Writing a scale from 1–10 on the board, with a smiling face for the number 10 and a frown for the number 1, allows even very young children to use scales effectively. Handing patients the marker and board, and asking them to circle the number they think they are at, concretely gives them the responsibility for their answer while positioning them in the role of expert. It communicates the importance of their input in the session, and places the responsibility for achieving their goals literally into their hands. It is a small but powerful intervention.

Patients learn to expect that scaling questions will be asked and frequently will come to an appointment offering to say where things are from 1–10, without even being asked. Children often write their own versions of the scale on the board and pretend to be a teacher. Scaling questions become fun for patients while reinforcing their ability to make choices and create solutions in their own life.

Yvonne Dolan has created a wonderful set of scaling questions asking patients to rate their satisfaction with the degree to which their problem is being solved from 1–10. Patients are asked, "Supposing 10 is you are satisfied that your problem has been solved and 1 is the opposite, where would you say you are now?" "What makes it not lower?" "What would it take to raise the number by one point?" The interesting point about these questions is that you don't need to know the details of the problem in order to work toward solutions (Y. Dolan, personal communication).

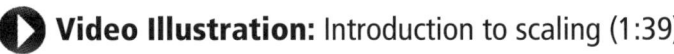 **Video Illustration:** Introduction to scaling (1:39)

Learning Exercise: Scaling

Ask a group participant to briefly describe, taking not more than 2 minutes, a problem he or she is having. It is recommended that the participant reveal a problem that is not too personal, given the nature of a group setting. Ask the participant to rate how satisfied he or she is that the problem has been solved from 1–10, where 10 is they are satisfied and 1 is the opposite. Begin by asking what makes the number not lower, and what else makes it not lower, until the participant is unable to detail any more successes. Then ask what it would take to move this number forward by one point, and what else it would take to move forward. Ask what a 10 would look like. Ask how the person's VIPs would rate how satisfied they are about the problem being solved. It is very interesting to see the myriad useful solutions that come out of these conversations, all without a lengthy discussion of the problem. You can then have the participants break up into groups of two and practice this exercise with each other.

Case Illustration: Scaling

Brittany was a 10-year-old girl who came in with her mother for a routine psychopharmacology session to monitor her medications. She was living with her mother and four siblings. Brittany was being treated for attention-deficit/hyperactivity disorder and a mood disorder. Her mother was also in treatment for a mood disorder. Their relationship had suffered from high conflict, parent and child mood instability, and parental stress. This excerpt begins after a conversation about what has been better. Several positive differences were identified, including that Brittany and her mother were not fighting as much, Brittany was working on stopping and thinking things through, and her mother was using a new point system at home. Her mother talked about how the point system helped them to stay on the same page so they could get along better. The excerpt begins at this point in the session and demonstrates how scaling can help defuse conflict while also maintaining the session in a goal-oriented direction.

ANNE: Suppose 10 is the two of you are on the same page, getting along and doing fun things together and 1 is the opposite, where would you say you are now?

It can be helpful to spend time amplifying positive differences prior to asking scaling questions. This often results in patients giving higher numbers. Just as with other solution-focused questions, it is essential to incorporate the patient's language within the question.

MOTHER: 4.

ANNE: And Brittany, where would you say you are at?

Scaling questions help both parent and child learn about each other's perspectives in a calm and nonconfrontational manner, piquing their curiosity in the other's response.

BRITTANY: 4.

ANNE: Is that number going up or down?

BRITTANY: Up. It used to be way lower.

ANNE: What makes that number not lower?

It is important to begin by asking what makes the number NOT lower. This digs for further positive relationship differences, strengthening the parent-child bond.

BRITTANY: We're drawing together. (*They were actually drawing a picture together in the room as they were answering these questions.*)

A positive difference is discovered.

ANNE: I can see you are creating a beautiful picture together. Is that different that you are drawing together?

When parents and children are doing something positive and productive together, it is important to compliment and explore this potential positive difference.

BRITTANY: Yes.

ANNE: How is that different?

BRITTANY: We would never do things that we both enjoy and that we have in common.

ANNE: Is it helpful for you to find things you both enjoy and have in common?

BRITTANY: Yes.

ANNE: How is it helpful for you to find things you both enjoy and have in common?

BRITTANY: We have more fun together and talk more. I feel closer to my mom.

More positive differences are discovered.

ANNE: That is fantastic how you are able to talk, enjoy things together, and feel closer. Are there other things you have found you enjoy and have in common together?

Direct compliments are furnished prior to exploring for more details of their relational success.

BRITTANY: We both like clothes and shopping.

ANNE: That's great. What else do you find in common?

I continue to amplify details of their success by asking what else they find in common.

BRITTANY: We like to play games. My mom played tag with us the other day.

ANNE: Wow! (*Looking at mom.*) You are doing a lot. Not every mom would play tag with her children. What do you think makes it not lower than a 4?

Asking what makes the number not lower amplifies more details of success.

MOTHER: She's right. We are drawing and doing more things that are fun for both of us. And she is listening more. That helps too.

ANNE: What else makes it not lower than a 4?

MOTHER: We're getting along better and not fighting. I am also working on my issues in my own therapy.

ANNE: I am impressed how hard you are both working. I wonder what you think it would take to make that number go up to a 5, just a little bit higher?

I bridge a compliment prior to asking what it would take to increase the number.

BRITTANY: If we went out shopping together.

MOTHER: Yes. She's right. That is the next step. I just get very anxious in big shopping malls. I'm trying to find smaller stores we can go to.

Realistic goals and next steps are agreed upon.

ANNE: I am impressed by the hard work you are both doing. I am wondering if I could challenge you to a task.

Framing a therapeutic homework task as a challenge instead of homework generally is more motivating to children. Most children are up for a challenge, and inviting them to participate in this challenge implies you have confidence that they will be successful.

BRITTANY: Yes. I like challenges.

ANNE: I am so impressed by all the new things you have discovered that you enjoy together. I am also impressed how hard you are both working at improving things at home; implementing point systems and finding things you both have in common. This will be difficult to do, but I am wondering if you could both pay attention to times when you think things are a 5 between the two of you, just a little bit better.

Scaling questions can also be used as tools to help patients notice differently, and can be offered as suggestions or homework.

BRITTANY: Sure.

Video Illustration: Scaling the next step (1:53)

Scaling Without a Description of the Problem

There are times, especially in working with children, when the child does not want to talk about the problem but the parent is bursting at the seams to express concern about the child's difficulties. Scaling questions can be extremely useful in these circumstances. The following illustration demonstrates how scaling questions can be used to negotiate goals without needing a detailed description of the problem.

Case Illustration: Scaling Without the Problem

Katie was a 13-year-old girl being treated for anxiety. She came to a routine follow-up appointment. The session began with a discussion of what had been better. She was able to talk about her schoolwork and said she was managing much better with her assignment notebook. She was remembering to bring it with her to all her classes, write down the homework assignments, and then do what was asked. Her mother was pleased with her progress and rated how well she was doing her homework as an 8 out of 10, but then wanted to talk about problems and concerns she had about her daughter. Katie was adamant that her mother not speak about them, while her mother was trying to get help for her daughter. The following is an excerpt from this portion of the session demonstrating how to use scaling questions in these situations.

KATIE: I don't want you to talk about that. All you do is bring up the bad stuff. Why do you need to do this now, after we just talked about good things?

ANNE: Of course, I can see how upsetting this is for you. I am wondering if you could help me by just answering a few number questions. I won't directly ask you about the problem. I call it the prediction game. Would this be something you would be willing to play?

I acknowledge Katie's concerns by providing an emotional yes-set "for you" response, and then bridge this by asking if she could help me, not her mother, by answering a few number questions. Asking children if they would be willing to answer a number question and play a game is generally more inviting for them. They then usually agree to this conversational step.

KATIE: OK.

ANNE: Suppose I have a number from 1–10, where 10 is your mother is satisfied that the problem you came here with was solved and 1 is the opposite, where do you think your mother would rate things for you now?

KATIE: I don't know.

ANNE: Of course, this must be a difficult question for you. Let me start by asking your mother where she thinks things are.

I decide to not push Katie at this point. She has at least agreed to participate in the conversation, so I decide to pursue her mother's perspective.

MOTHER: A 4.

ANNE: And what makes the number not lower?

MOTHER: She does what I ask some of the time.

A positive difference has been identified and can be amplified.

ANNE: Is that helpful when she does that?

MOTHER: Yes.

ANNE: How is it helpful?

MOTHER: We have more time to do fun things and I don't get so irritated with her.

ANNE: How else is it helpful?

MOTHER: We get along better. The whole family is more relaxed.

ANNE: What would it take to raise it by one point?

I ask what would make it one point higher, only after an exploration of what makes it not lower.

MOTHER: If when I asked her to do something, she would say OK.

ANNE: I think that's one of a parent's favorite words. "OK" is a beautiful word (*smiling*). What else would make it one point higher?

MOTHER: She would just do what I ask without arguing. She wouldn't argue.

This is a very common response for parents, needing their children to say OK and do what is asked.

ANNE: Of course. And Katie, what do you think would make it one point higher?

I now try to get Katie's ideas of what would raise the number by one.

KATIE: I wouldn't argue with her.

She is able to answer, but gives her response in the negative.

ANNE: What would you do instead?

This question assists patients in formulating goals in positive language.

KATIE: I would say OK.

ANNE: I am impressed how you both agree on this. What else would make it one point higher?

KATIE: I would do what she asks right away.

As you can see, this brief conversation led to a productive discussion of solutions without a detailed discussion of the problem through the use of scaling questions. They both agreed on several useful ideas to move things forward without escalating conflict.

The Miracle Question

The miracle question is a unique question created by Insoo Kim Berg and Steve de Shazer in the 1980s (Berg 1994; de Shazer 1988). It is not simply a question, but a tool used to facilitate patients thinking about future possibilities when their problem is solved (Berg and de Shazer 1993; de Shazer et al. 2007). Yvonne Dolan has adapted this question by integrating a scaling question within it. It requires a great deal of imagination and is distinctive in requiring patients to envision their life without their presenting problem. This question helps patients to define their goals and illuminate solutions (Berg and de Shazer 1993). The following is a description of the miracle question (de Shazer 2000).

I know I have already asked a lot of questions, but I'm wondering if it would be ok to ask you a strange question that requires some imagination? This is probably the most difficult question I ask, and I know I ask many hard questions. (*Pause and wait for the client response.*) Suppose that tonight after you have done your usual things and have finally fallen asleep, a miracle happens. The miracle is that while you were sleeping, the problems that brought you here are solved, but because you were sleeping, you didn't know that it happened. (*Pause.*) So, when you wake up in the morning, the miracle has happened and you experience a 10 day. What do you suppose would be the first thing you would notice that would tell you a miracle 10 day has happened, and the problem that brought you here is solved?

This question can be adapted for young children who do not yet understand what a miracle is. The version of the miracle question for young children is called the *fairy godmother/magic wand question.* Instead of asking the child to imagine a miracle, the clinician brings out a magic wand. The wand is a toy filled with brightly colored stars, moons, and sparkles. Children are shown the wand, and told they can play with it after they try and answer this difficult question. This toy is hidden away from the regular toys and becomes especially intriguing to them. Asking children whether they have a good imagination conveys they will need this skill to answer the question. Preparing children in this way facilitates them answering this important question. The following is a description of the fairy godmother/magic wand question.

The Fairy Godmother/Magic Wand Question

Imagine after you go through your usual day, you go to bed. And while you are sleeping, your fairy godmother comes and sprinkles this magic dust over your pillow and makes all your problems go away. When you wake up you are having a 10 day. But the stars, sprinkles, and moons from the wand disappear from your pillow so you cannot see them when you wake up in the morning. As you are going through you day, what would tell you that your fairy godmother came, and your day is a 10?

The miracle/magic wand question transforms the patient's attention from the presenting problem to a problem that is solved (Pichot and Smock 2009). If the question is posed in terms of a miracle, patients do not have to be concerned with how their goals will be achieved, but instead focus on how their lives will be different when the miracle occurs. This removes their anxiety about how they will have to produce the solution, and instead facilitates a more detailed description of their preferred solution or best hopes for their future. This question allows patients the freedom to think beyond the problems that seem insurmountable and allows them to identify resources that they may not remember or recognize when their minds are clouded by the problem. Children and adults alike love surprises. A miracle is most often perceived as a positive surprise with huge ramifications. Perceiving it as a miracle ensures that the change will be worthwhile to them and not something that they could have easily obtained without assistance. Another component of the miracle question is that the miracle occurs *tonight.* This creates a sense of immediacy, as well as hope that change may occur right away (Pichot and Smock 2009). It empowers patients to search for hints of change right away, in the session with you. Telling patients that they are not aware the miracle occurred during the night encourages them to work hard at discovering what will be different when their "miracle 10 day" does occur. The questions shown in Table 5–2 are follow-up questions that assist patients in discovering clues that would tell them their miracle 10 day has happened.

TABLE 5–2.   Follow-up questions to the miracle question

- What will be the first thing you notice when you are lying in bed that would tell you your "miracle 10 day" happened?
- What else will you notice before you get up?
- What will you notice you are doing differently as you go through your day?
- What else will you be doing differently on your miracle 10 day?
- What will your VIPs notice you doing differently that would tell them your miracle 10 day happened?
- What else would your VIPs notice that you were doing differently on your miracle 10 day?
- What will be different between you and your VIPs when your miracle 10 day happens?
- What else would be different between you and your VIPs?
- On a scale of 1–10, where 10 is the day after the miracle, and 1 is the opposite, where would you say you are now?
- What makes the number not lower?
- What else would make it not lower?
- What would it take to raise it by one point?
- Where do you think your VIPs would rate you?
- What would tell your VIPs that the number rose one point?
- What else would they notice you doing when the number rises one point?

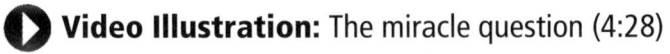 **Video Illustration:** The miracle question (4:28)

Case Illustration: The Fairy Godmother/Magic Wand Question

James was a 5-year-old boy who was recently hospitalized after threatening to kill himself with a knife. He had child protective services involved for several years because of concerns about his parents' abilities to care for him. James had suffered a complicated past. His biological father broke James's arm when he was 2 years old. His mother had experienced domestic violence, and she suffered from PTSD as well as from depression that had required several psychiatric hospitalizations; she also had been in foster care as a child and adolescent. She separated from her son's father after the trauma of her son's broken arm. His mother desperately wanted to get her son back home with her. James had been diagnosed with PTSD and attachment difficulties. In the past he had received trials of several stimulants, none of which were helpful. He came to an outpatient appointment with his foster father and biological mother. Child protective services were requiring a diagnostic and medication evaluation. The following is an excerpt from the middle of his initial session, demonstrating the fairy godmother/ magic wand question.

ANNE: I would like to show you something special. (*I pull out a magic wand from my desk drawer.*) Do you have a pretty good imagination? (*James nods yes.*) This is a pretend magic wand. It is filled with stars and moons. Would you like to hold it? (*He nods affirmatively.*) You are welcome to hold it after you try your best to answer this difficult question.

JAMES: Can't I hold it now?

ANNE: Of course you will be able to hold it, but first I would like you to try and answer this question. Would that be OK?

Waiting to give James the magic wand after he tries to answer the question helps to maintain his motivation.

JAMES: OK.

ANNE: Do you know what a fairy godmother is?

JAMES: Yes. It's kind of like a tooth fairy.

ANNE: Exactly, you are very smart. Imagine that when you go to sleep tonight and while are sleeping, your fairy godmother comes. She comes and sprinkles this magic dust on your pillow (*showing him the wand*). This dust is special and makes all your worries and problems go away. When you wake up, the dust is gone and so are your worries and problems. You are having a 10 day. What do you imagine you would be doing after she came at night that would tell you that your problems were gone and you were having a 10 day?

MOTHER: That question is too hard for him.

ANNE: You're right. This is a very difficult question and it may be too hard for him, but your son is very smart and I think we should give it a try. James, what do you think would tell you your worries were gone, and you were having a 10 day when you woke up in the morning?

Rather than argue with her, I agree, maintaining the yes-set. By continuing in my pursuit of this question, I am conveying an expectation that James will rise to the challenge. Framing the question as very difficult will help him save face, if he genuinely cannot answer it, or give him a boost of confidence while making his mother proud, if he does.

JAMES: My bad thoughts wouldn't be there.

ANNE: What do you mean "bad thoughts"?

JAMES: My scary dreams.

ANNE: Those must be scary for you. When your 10 day happens, what would there be instead of bad thoughts?

Patients often answer with what would not be there (i.e., no bad thoughts). It is important to help patients figure out what they would be "doing instead."

JAMES: Nice things.

ANNE: What nice things would you be doing?

While this is a start in terms of being more positive, it is still rather vague and requires detailing what he would be "doing."

JAMES: I would take a boat ride with my mother.

He is able to articulate a positive, measurable goal that may also help his mother realize what he needs from her.

ANNE: I can see you really like to spend time with your mother. What other nice things would you do with your mother when the bad thoughts are gone?

Underscoring his desire to spend time with his mother provides an indirect compliment to his mother, highlighting a positive aspect of their bond. This is paired with a question that gathers more details of what they can do together, focusing on strengthening their relationship.

JAMES: I would play with her.

ANNE: What would you play with her?

JAMES: We would go to the park.

ANNE: What else would you do with your mother?

JAMES: I would be good.

ANNE: What do you do when you are good?

JAMES: I don't get into trouble. (*He is now appearing more restless.*)

ANNE: Wow! You have done a great job answering this question. Not many 5-year-olds could answer such a hard question. You are very smart. (*I now hand him the magic wand.*) Mom, where does he get this ability?

His restlessness indicates it may be time to end this difficult line of questioning. I provide a direct compliment to him, followed by an indirect compliment to his mother. Asking children where they get their abilities from conveys parental competencies.

MOTHER: Me! (*Laughing.*)

She laughs and is able to appreciate her own strength.

ANNE: Of course, I can see that. I am wondering, Mom, what would tell you that the fairy godmother came and James was having a 10 day? What would you notice he was doing differently?

I now begin to explore his mother's vision of the miracle/magic wand question. Exploring a patient's VIP's picture of the miracle further enhances the vision of their preferred future, simultaneously helping them set goals together.

MOTHER: He would listen and be happy. All I want is for him to be happy.

ANNE: I can see how much you care about your son. What would he be doing that would tell you he is happy?

I need to clarify the meaning of "happy" by asking what he would be "doing" when he is happy.

MOTHER: He wouldn't have all these meltdowns or hurt himself.

ANNE: What would he be doing instead of hurting himself or having meltdowns?

MOTHER: He would listen and do what I say at least some of the time.

ANNE: What else would he be doing when he is happy?

MOTHER: We would go to the park or the store together.

The session continued, and both James and his mother were asked scaling questions. They were asked, supposing 10 was the day after your fairy godmother came and 1 was the opposite, where would they say things are now? James was given a magic marker and circled the number 7. Mother also gave him a 7. These numbers provided opportunities to ask what made the number not lower and what it would take to raise it by one point.

This vignette illustrates how the miracle/magic wand question helps to clarify goals for both the child and parent, while at the same time enhancing treatment alliance. As can be seen from this vignette, asking detailed follow-up questions to the miracle/fairy godmother/magic wand question is critical in negotiating the patient's goals. The miracle/magic wand question is in essence a question that helps patients clarify their goals.

Scaling questions are a methodical technique to use after the miracle/magic wand question has been asked. They sustain the conversation toward the patient's goals and best hopes for his or her preferred future. This will be discussed further in the next chapter, on solution-focused goal negotiation.

▶ **Video Illustration:** Scaling the miracle (3:54)

▶ **Video Illustration:** Scaling the miracle with a child (1:54)

KEY POINTS

- Scaling questions are self-anchored rather than normed. The patient, not the clinician, defines what the numbers mean.
- Scaling questions are not used to measure the extent of the problem, but rather the scope of the solution.
- Scaling questions can quickly and metaphorically bring the patient's VIPs [very important people] into the office.
- Scaling questions can be used to amplify ambivalence in externally motivated patients.
- Asking how things are "between" a patient and the patient's VIPs quickly assesses the health of these important relationships.
- Asking what makes the number not lower amplifies hope, confidence, and successes.
- Asking what it takes to raise it by one point helps negotiate goals.
- The miracle question is a tool used to help patients imagine their preferred future when their problem is solved.
- It is critical to follow up the miracle question with further questions, including scaling questions, that detail this vision.
- Asking a patient what his or her VIPs would notice when the miracle happens broadens the vision to include the patient's social context.

References

Berg IK: Family Based Services: A Solution-Focused Approach. New York, WW Norton, 1994

Berg IK, de Shazer S: Making Numbers Talk: Language in Therapy, in The New Language of Change: Constructive Collaboration in Psychotherapy. Edited by Friedman S. New York, Guilford, 1993, pp 5–24

de Shazer S: Clues: Investigating Solutions in Brief Therapy. New York, NY, WW Norton, 1988

de Shazer S: The Miracle Question. BFTC—Brief Family Therapy Center, 2000. Available at: http://www.netzwerk-ost.at/publikationen/pdf/miraclequestion.pdf. Accessed February 20, 2013.

de Shazer S, Dolan Y, Korman H, et al: More Than Miracles: The State of the Art of Solution-Focused Brief Therapy. New York, Haworth, 2007

Pichot T, Smock SA: Solution-Focused Substance Abuse Treatment. New York, Routledge/Taylor & Francis Group, 2009

Pilowsky DJ, Wickramaratne P, Talati A, et al: Children of depressed mothers 1 year after the initiation of maternal treatment: findings from the STAR*D-Child Study. Am J Psychiatry 165:1136–1147, 2008

Weissman MM, Pilowsky DJ, Wickramaratne PJ, et al: Remissions in maternal depression and child psychopathology: a STAR*D-child report. JAMA 295:1389–1398, 2006

Wickramaratne P, Gameroff MJ, Pilowsky DJ, et al: Children of depressed mothers 1 year after remission of maternal depression: findings from the STAR*D-Child study. Am J Psychiatry 168:593–602, 2011

CHAPTER 6

Solution-Focused Goal Negotiation

General Principles in Goal Negotiation

Negotiating goals with patients is an essential skill in solution-focused therapy. Solution-focused therapy concentrates intensely on developing well-formed goals with patients (De Jong and Miller 1995). In all forms of therapy, both the clinician and the patient work on establishing criteria that tell them when they have succeeded and can end therapy. This necessitates collaboratively developing criteria for success. It is one thing to know where you don't want to be, but quite another to know where you want to go instead. Negotiating goals with patients helps define the direction of treatment, determines whether treatment is successful, and strengthens the treatment alliance.

In medicine, goal negotiation involves asking patients about their chief complaint. "Why are you here today?" is the standard question often asked by physicians when beginning an interview. The solution-focused clinician asks different questions, in a different order. The solution-focused clinician begins the query with where patients want to go in their life and their best hopes for their preferred future, rather than what problems brought them in to seek help. This chapter will describe how a solution-focused clinician negotiates the goals and tasks of therapy.

The first step in goal negotiation is to identify and broaden areas of agreement. Amplifying patients' competencies as described in previous chapters, including their relationship resources through the exploration of their very important people (VIPs), is the crucial first step in successful goal negotiation. It is generally easier to agree on things that people are good at, that they enjoy, that are important to them, and that are going well than on areas of conflict and disagreement. Building areas of agreement through the identification and amplification of positive differences provides meta-phorical conversational "deposits" for the forthcoming dialog.

Goal negotiation is difficult enough when one person is involved in the process, but for clinicians working with multiple people, such as families, couples, and systems, goal negotiation becomes all the more challenging be-cause of the need to simultaneously negotiate goals with the myriad people involved in a patient's life, many of whom may have very different and con-flicting agendas. This can be especially challenging in working with exter-nally motivated patients who do not perceive there is any problem, even while their VIPs are desperate to talk about their loved one's problems. Table 6–1 lists some of the basic questions that clinicians ask in order to collabora-tively negotiate goals with patients. These questions will be elaborated on in this chapter.

Learning solution-focused therapy requires steering conversations to-ward what one's patients' best hopes and aspirations are for their lives. In-viting patients to imagine a future time without the problem and then work backwards is a very different and unfamiliar process for most people. Peo-ple who are in distress and have many problems are naturally inclined to talk about the painful things in their life. Inviting patients to imagine their best hopes for their future does not mean ignoring their feelings of pain and frustration with how their life is currently proceeding. It is essential to provide empathic responses for the difficult and painful experiences they may be feeling by providing enough "for you" responses, termed in previ-ous chapters the *emotional yes-set*. It is also critical to provide enough com-pliments, both direct and indirect, through the amplification of positive differences. There is no arguing about what patients are good at or what their emotional experience is for them. Pairing "for you" statements and compliments with solution-focused questions is critical when helping pa-tients negotiate goals.

After enough time has been spent building patient competencies through the identification and amplification of positive differences, evalu-ating a patient's VIPs, building a yes-set, and providing compliments, it is then time to begin goal negotiation. Goal negotiation begins with ques-tions that encourage patients to imagine what their life would be like with-out the problem, rather than a direct and deep exploration of their difficulties. This is no small task. People are often more familiar talking about what they don't want in their life, rather than what things will look like when their problem is solved. Learning solution-focused therapy re-quires becoming a conversational guide helping patients clarify what they do want in their life, what they will be doing instead of their problematic

---

TABLE 6–1.   Solution-focused goal negotiation questions

Questions for motivated patients

- What are your "best hopes" for coming to this appointment so this meeting will be helpful for you?
- How can I be most helpful "for you" today so this meeting is useful for you and you can say it was worthwhile coming to see me?
- What have you tried so far that has been helpful?
- What else have you tried?
- What will you be "doing instead" of your problematic behavior?
- What else would you be "doing instead"?
- What are your best hopes for a medication?
- Supposing there was a magic pill (which we know there is not), what are your best hopes for how a medication will be helpful for you?
- What do you need?
- What else do you need?
- The miracle question/magic wand question, as described in Chapter 5.
- What would be different between you and your VIPs when the problematic behaviors no longer are occurring?
- What else would be different between you and your VIPs when the problematic behaviors are no longer occurring?
- Supposing 10 is you are satisfied that your problem is solved and 1 is the opposite: where would you say things are now?
- What makes this number not lower?
- What would it take to raise it by one point?

Questions for externally motivated patients

- Whose idea was it for you to come here today?
- What were they concerned about that they thought it might be helpful for you to come here today?
- What needs to happen for your VIPs to get off your back?
- What do your VIPs need to see you do so you don't have to come here anymore?
- How does your VIP know you can do this?
- How confidently would your VIP say you can do this?
- On a scale of 1–10, where 10 is your VIPs no longer think you need to come here and 1 is the opposite, what number do you suppose they would give you?
- What do your VIPs need from you?
- What else do your VIPs need from you?

---

behavior, and what will be different between them and their VIPs when their problem is solved (Berg 1994; De Jong and Berg 2002).

Qualities of Well-formed Goals

Well-formed goals have several key features (De Jong and Berg 2002). An important quality of well-formed goals is that they must be important to the patient and viewed as personally beneficial. Unless the goal is important to the patient, he or she will have difficulties investing in all the hard work it will take to accomplish it. Beginning the conversation with what the person's best hopes are, and how you could be most helpful so the meeting is worthwhile for him or her maintains the focus on what is most important for the patient.

Well-formed goals are described in relational and contextual terms. This requires knowledge of a patient's VIPs. A patient's VIPs are the social context in which they must develop their solutions (de Shazer 1988). Recall that for problems to get solved, both the patient and his or her VIPs must no longer view the behavior as problematic. Incorporating a patient's VIPs within the conversation helps to broaden the perspective of problems and solutions to see them through the eyes of others who are most important in the patient's life. This can generate many possibilities. This is important for all people, but especially so in working with children and adolescents, who are often externally motivated. VIPs, both acknowledged (e.g., parents), and hidden (e.g., probation officers) are important to incorporate into the conversation when negotiating goals. Patients live and spend their lives in a variety of social contexts with many different people who are important to them, including parents, children, siblings, primary caretakers, friends, grandparents, teachers, coaches, and cousins, to name a few. Incorporating a patient's VIPs within goal negotiation questions can help the patient better articulate goals, amplify ambivalence, and uncover further possibilities for solutions.

▶ **Video Illustration:** Goal negotiation and exploring best hopes (3:01)

Strategies for Coping With the "I Don't Know" Response

Particularly with children, adolescents, and externally motivated patients, there are times when their reply to solution-focused questions is "I don't know." Several strategies can help handle the "I don't know" response. In these situations, it can be helpful to integrate the patient's VIPs into the question. Asking adolescents what their parent is "worried" about that made the parent think it would be a good idea "for you" to come and see the clinician is one method to engage them in goal negotiation. This invites their perspective to shift from what they are doing wrong to how concerned their parent is about them. When patients respond to questions with "I don't know," this can also mean they need more time to think about the difficult question posed to them. Becoming comfortable with pauses in the conversation, taking responsibility for the difficult questions asked, and validating patients' need to take more time to think about the challenging questions that you have posed often results in a thoughtful answer. Usually after a pause patients are able to respond, especially if enough time has been spent building competencies, providing conversational deposits, strengthening relationships through the VIP line of questioning, and furnishing plenty of compliments. Another question that can be helpful when patients respond with "I don't know" is to ask them the following: "Suppose you did know, what would you be doing?" This question often helps patients to think differently about the question and keeps the conversational ball in their court.

Well-formed goals must be realistic, specific, and small enough to be achieved. They are described in positive behavioral terms as the presence, rather than the absence, of something. A well-formed goal is stated in proactive language about what the patient will do versus what he or she will not do (Berg and Miller 1992). The verb *to do* is a powerful one used frequently in solution-focused goal negotiation questions. Let's recall the quintessential idea in becoming solution focused. When things are working, do more of them, and when they are not, do something different (de Shazer 1990). Recollect that people solve problems by doing something differently. Incorporating the verb *doing* within questions linguistically assists patients in formulating well-formed goals. When patients describe their goals in vague and negative behavioral terms, such as not wanting to feel so depressed, specific questions (as shown in Table 6–2) can help clarify their goals in small, realistic, action-oriented ways. Notice how the word *do* is incorporated into these questions.

When patients are asked what they most want help with, they frequently answer with negatively stated goals. They may say they don't want to feel depressed, don't want to feel anxious, don't want the school to call every day because their child is getting into trouble, or don't want to fight with their spouse. In these situations, it is helpful to ask what Insoo Kim Berg termed the "doing instead" question (Berg and Miller 1992). This question asks what patients will be doing instead of their negatively stated behaviors. Humans are always in a state of doing something, and even when apparently doing nothing are doing something, such as sitting, med-

TABLE 6–2.	**Questions using "to do" to help clarify goals**

- What will you be doing instead when you are no longer feeling so depressed?
- What will you be doing differently when you are happy?
- What else will you be doing?
- What will your VIPs notice you doing when you are happy?
- Supposing you wake up on a Saturday morning and look back at your week and say, "Wow, that was a great week." During a great week, what do you suppose you would be doing?
- What else would you be doing?
- What would your VIPs notice you doing?

itating, thinking, or sleeping. Asking patients what they will be *doing instead* guides the conversation toward positively stated and action-oriented goals.

Describing goals in precise, positive, and action-oriented terms allows the clinician and patient to better evaluate treatment progress. Establishing goals in small, concrete, and behavioral steps can be a painstaking process for the solution-focused clinician, especially when patients respond to questions with "I don't know" or persist in stating their goals in negative behavioral terms. It takes persistence on the part of the clinician to sustain the query in ways that prompt patients to restate their goals in positive behavioral terms. Asking what they will be doing instead or doing differently is the linguistic question that directs a patient's goals in positive, small, realistic, and, most important, action-oriented ways. Persisting in efforts to ask patients what they will be doing instead of their problematic behaviors often yields myriad positive behaviors. For example, when parents are asked what their children will be doing instead of various problematic behaviors, responses may include that they will smile more, get up more easily in the morning, get their chores done with less arguing, clean their room, do more fun things together with the family, get their homework done, be more involved with friends, come out of their room more often, talk more, and get along better with the family. When clinicians persist in asking children what they will do instead of their problematic behaviors, they often respond by saying they will get up more easily in the morning, get ready for school, do their work at school, get along with others, stay out of trouble, pass to the next grade, ignore disruptive peers, listen to their teachers, talk things through, ask for help, get their homework done, and say OK to their parents' demands. When parents and children are asked what they will be doing differently when they are not arguing, they often respond by talking about how they will be getting along better with each other, doing more things together, talking more, and having more time to do fun things together.

What Have They Tried?

Another useful question to ask patients while negotiating goals with them is to inquire about what they have tried to do to solve their problem or cope with their difficulties. These questions convey to patients your respect and your faith that they have been working hard at solving their problems. Asking what they have already tried to do to help often uncovers additional resources that had not yet been identified. It also prevents the clinician from giving unsolicited advice about steps that patients have already taken to try to help themselves. Asking what else they tried continues the pursuit of strengths and resources.

 Video Illustration: "What have you tried?" (1:57)

The word *skill* is an important one in negotiating goals with patients (Furman 2011). All people enjoy learning new skills. Many people, especially children, also enjoy challenges. All people want to be seen as normal, want to be accepted as part of a social group, and enjoy the challenge of learning new skills. Asking patients whether they are up to the challenge of learning new skills such as calming down, listening, focusing, asking for help, or getting along better with adults reframes their goals as challenges and as skill building. This enhances their motivation, while communicating that the clinician has confidence in their potential to rise to the challenge of learning new skills.

When Patients See Their Problems as Someone Else's Fault

It is not unusual for patients to see their problems as being someone else's fault. For example: spouses may complain that if only their partner would change, everything would be solved; children may think it is someone else's fault that they are getting into trouble; workers may say, "If my boss wasn't so bad, my job would be great." When patients think the solution of their problems lies in someone else's hands, the clinician's challenge is to guide the conversation toward what patients can do to solve their problems and meet their goals. The solution-focused clinician approaches this dilemma with the following question.

> Suppose (X) wouldn't do (problematic behavior) anymore; what would "you be doing" instead (or differently) when that happens?

Let's look closely at this question with an example.

"If Tommy wouldn't annoy me so much, I wouldn't hit him."

Using the algorithm above, one possible response would be to ask:

"Suppose Tommy wouldn't annoy you so much, what would you be doing instead of hitting him?"

The first word, *suppose*, combined with the exact wording of the patient, invites him to imagine a different and contrasting scenario. Incorporating the patient's words, that "Tommy wouldn't annoy [me] so much," builds a shared dialect between patient and clinician. This statement is then bridged by asking what the patient would "be doing" *when* (not *if*) the problematic behavior no longer occurs, "*instead of* hit[ting] him"—again incorporating his exact words. Using the word *when*, not *if*, compels the patient to think about an alternative possibility to the current problematic state of affairs. This redirects the conversation toward what he can "do instead" to change and control the situation, increasing his sense of self-efficacy. Solution-focused language often incorporates presuppositional language within the questions that are asked. Presuppositional language imbeds part of the solution within the questions asked (O'Hanlon and Weiner-Davis 1989). This invites patients to surmise, conjecture, speculate, hypothesize, postulate, and have hunches. A suppositional query asks questions that allow people to imagine an alternate reality, different from their current situation. These types of questions inspire creativity, inventiveness, imagination, and resourcefulness in children and adults alike.

Well-formed goals are described as a beginning rather than an end. As it is often said, the journey of a thousand miles begins with a single step. Helping patients think about what first small steps they will need to take to move toward their goals and asking them what it would take to get to the next level are two questions that can help them stay focused on doable next small steps. Patients who move toward their goals in a step-by-step fashion are more likely to accomplish them. Scaling questions are extremely helpful in keeping patients focused on the next small next steps to reach their goals (Berg and de Shazer 1993). For example, when a parent and an adolescent want to have a better relationship with each other, it can be difficult to define what this will look like in realistic terms. Asking both the parent and the adolescent to rate how things are "between" the two of them from 1–10, where 10 is the best and 1 the opposite, helps to more clearly define their goals in realistic terms. The usual line of scaling questions follows by asking what makes the number not lower, what else makes it not lower, and what it would take to raise it by one point.

Well-formed goals are perceived as hard work by patients. Conveying to patients how much effort it will take to move toward their goals assists them in internalizing and taking responsibility and credit for achieving their aims. At the same time, framing goals in this way provides a face-saving function should they be unable to achieve their goal (Berg 1994). Declaring that the goal will be hard work and difficult to achieve makes a point that can easily be agreed upon, and emphasizing this point validates the patient's efforts. If the patient is unable to meet the goal, the clinician can agree, validate, and normalize that the goal is very challenging and that it makes sense that more work is understandably required. If the patient achieves the goal, it can be an opportunity to compliment him or her on succeeding and to give the patient all the credit for the accomplishment.

▶ **Video Illustration:** Goal negotiation with an externally motivated patient (2:36)

Case Illustration: Goal Negotiation Using the Miracle Question

Kelly was a 15-year-old girl who was referred for a consultation because of concerns about depression and anxiety. She described escalating irritability, anxiety, and panic symptoms occurring for the past month. She lived with her mother and father, both hard-working and very concerned about her. Her mother worked in banking and her father was a counselor. Kelly was bright and herself very hard-working. The session began by making conversational deposits through an exploration of her strengths, her VIPs, and what she most appreciated about her VIPs. She talked about her skills in babysitting, her desire to work with young children and become a kindergarten teacher, and her positive choices in life and nonuse of drugs and alcohol. She talked about the ways she appreciated her parents and how they were people she could always go and talk with and get support from. She also talked about the other important people in her life, including her siblings and teachers at her school. Her parents talked about their daughter's caring and empathetic nature, how others did not sway her, how she worked hard and did very well in school. Kelly described her moods as like a light switch that would go on and off. When she felt more depressed and anxious, she would isolate herself in her room, avoid spending time with friends and family, stop eating, lose weight, and disconnect from the world around her. In the past, she had tried cutting herself to cope with her emotional pain. Her mother reported that Kelly has suffered from anxiety for many years, with her first concerns being at age 7 years. The following is an excerpt from an initial session taken at the point when she was asked the miracle question.

ANNE: I am now going to ask probably the most difficult question I ask, and I ask many hard questions. It is a strange question that requires a lot of imagination. Would you be willing to give it a try?

KELLY: Yes.

ANNE: Suppose that after you go through your day and do your usual things, you then go to bed. During the middle of the night while you are sleeping, a miracle happens and all your problems, worries, and anxiety go away. Your day becomes a 10 on a scale of 1–10. But because you were asleep, you did not know that it happened. When you wake up in the morning and this miracle has happened, what would tell you things are different as you are lying in your bed and going through your day?

This miracle question was asked integrating a scaling question within the query.

KELLY: I wouldn't feel as anxious or depressed.

Her goals are negatively stated and vague.

ANNE: What would you be doing instead when you are feeling less anxious and depressed?

I ask a "doing instead" question, integrating her exact words.

KELLY: I wouldn't worry or think as much.

She continues to answer with negative goals.

ANNE: What would you be doing instead of worrying or thinking as much?

KELLY: I would be thinking that it's going to be a good day.

She now answers with a positive response, good day, but this response still remains vague.

ANNE: What would you be doing differently when it is a good day?

KELLY: I would be out of my room more.

Now she has finally come up with a concrete and specific behavior.

ANNE: What else would you be doing that would tell you it is a good day?

It is important to amplify details of positively stated goals by asking "what else."

KELLY: I would hang out with my friends and not feel like I need to go to someone all the time for help.

ANNE: What would you be doing instead of going to someone for help all the time?

KELLY: I wouldn't focus on the negative so much.

ANNE: What would you be doing instead of focusing on the negative?

This query takes persistence.

KELLY: I would focus more on the positive and have more fun doing things.

ANNE: What kind of fun things would you be doing?

Amplifying details of things she would be doing for fun.

KELLY: I would hang out more with my friends.

ANNE: What else would you be doing when you are having more fun?

KELLY: Maybe try out for a sports team.

ANNE: What kind of sports teams?

KELLY: I've thought about softball and track, but never have actually tried out for them.

ANNE: What would it take for you to try out for one of these teams?

KELLY: They have these teams at school. Several of my friends have been encouraging me to try out. I just need to go and do it.

ANNE: That's a great idea! What else would you be doing that would be fun for you?

I compliment her good idea and then continue to pursue more details of what it would like for her to do more fun things in her life.

KELLY: I'm in chorus and singing.

New information was revealed through the painstaking persistence of asking "what else" questions.

ANNE: Wow, that's great! Do you enjoy singing?

KELLY: Yes. I actually have performed in a quartet this year.

A potential positive difference is revealed and will be amplified.

ANNE: Is that different that you have performed in a quartet like this?

 Video Illustration: Scaling goals (2:59)

End-of-Session Feedback/Homework

End-of-session feedback or homework includes complimenting patients by recapping the positive differences discovered, noticing when things are better, doing more of what works, and paying attention to when things go up one point on their identified scale. Taking notes during the session, while paying particular attention to positive differences, can be extremely useful because it can be easy to forget details of the positive differences identified. After the portion of dialog noted above in the case illustration, the conversation ended with the clinician complimenting the patient on things such as her intelligence, her openness to get help, her skill at ignoring negative comments of peers and focusing on positives, her courage in singing in a quartet despite her anxiety, her desire to try out for sports teams, her ability to connect with so many people, and the fact that so many people care about her. This was then followed by a suggestion that she pay attention to when things are a 5, just a little bit better than the number 4, which is where she had rated herself at the present time in terms of her miracle. She was also encouraged to do more of those things that she noticed were helping her. End-of-session feedback helps patients prioritize what is working and what small steps to focus on in order to move forward toward their goals.

 Video Illustration: End-of-session feedback (1:37)

LEARNING EXERCISE: GOAL NEGOTIATION

Break up into groups of three, with one person acting as a patient, one person acting as a clinician, and one person acting as the observer. Have the clinician practice asking what the patient's best hopes are for treatment that, if fulfilled, would tell the patient the treatment was useful. Practice asking the "doing instead" question and scaling the patient's self-rating in relation to the goals and what it would take to move this up by one point. Have the observer log solution-focused questions that were asked. Have each member switch roles and discuss what this experience was like for them.

KEY POINTS

- Goal negotiation begins by building areas of agreement, amplifying positive differences, and exploring a patient's VIPs (very important people).

- Solution-focused goal negotiation focuses on patients' best hopes for their preferred future rather than the problems that brought them into treatment.

- In negotiating goals with externally motivated patients, it is important to know and integrate their VIPs within the goal negotiation questions.

- Well-formed goals are those that are important to the patient and that the patient views as personally beneficial.

- Well-formed goals are described in positive behavioral terms as the presence rather than the absence of something.

- Asking patients what they will be "doing instead" or "doing differently" directs a patient's goals in positive, action-oriented ways.

- Asking patients what they have tried to do to solve their problems that has helped often uncovers additional resources that were as yet unidentified.

- Scaling questions help to keep patients focused on small and realistic next steps needed to accomplish their goals.

- The miracle question is a powerful goal negotiation question.

- End-of-session feedback includes listing the positive differences identified in the form of compliments and encouraging patients to pay attention to what is working, do more of what is working, and pay attention to when a goal-related rating goes up by one point.

References

Berg IK: Family Based Services: A Solution-Focused Approach. New York, WW Norton, 1994

Berg IK, Miller SD: Working With the Problem Drinker: A Solution-Focused Approach. New York, WW Norton, 1992

Berg IK, de Shazer S: Making Numbers Talk: Language in Therapy, in The New Language of Change: Constructive Collaboration in Psychotherapy. Edited by Friedman S. New York, Guilford, 1993, pp 5–24

De Jong P, Berg IK: Interviewing for Solutions. Pacific Grove, CA, Brooks/Cole, 2002

De Jong P, Miller SD: How to interview for client strengths. Soc Work 40:729–736, 1995

de Shazer S: Clues: Investigating Solutions in Brief Therapy. New York, WW Norton, 1988

de Shazer S: What is it about brief therapy that works? in Brief Therapy: Myths, Methods, and Metaphors. Edited by Zeig JK, Gilligan SG. Philadelphia, PA, Brunner/Mazel, 1990, pp 90–99

Furman B: Kids' skills: an innovative and playful way to help children overcome problems. Educating Young Children: Learning and Teaching in the Early Childhood Years 17:24–27, 2011

O'Hanlon WH, Weiner-Davis M: In Search of Solutions: A New Direction in Psychotherapy. New York, WW Norton, 1989

CHAPTER 7

Other Useful
Solution-Focused Questions

This chapter will discuss several other questions that are useful in solution-focused therapy. These questions can be divided into four main categories: 1) those that are used in follow-up sessions, 2) those that are used in times of distress or crisis and when things are worse, 3) those that dig for details of success, and 4) those that amplify ambivalence.

Solution-Focused Follow-Up Sessions: What's Better?

A solution-focused follow-up session begins by asking patients "what is better" since the last meeting. This question is simple yet powerful. Commencing the interview by asking what's better immediately compels the patient to think about *what* has been better, not *if* anything has been better. They are obliged to consider positive differences in their life. Asking what is better is especially effective in work with children and adolescents, who are more likely to answer questions that bring into focus their skills, talents, and accomplishments. Asking "what else is better" expounds these attributes. Asking what their VIPs (very important people) notice is better reveals additional positive differences, expanding the possibility of developing further solutions. These newly discovered positive differences are then amplified by using the same series of questions exemplified throughout the book, beginning with: Was this different? How was it different? Was it helpful? How was it helpful? How did you do it? Were things different between others because of this difference? In solution-focused therapy there is an acronym, <u>EARS</u>, that illustrates this process: **E** for eliciting a positive difference or exception, **A** for amplifying this difference, **R** for reinforcing this difference, and **S** for starting the process over again when another positive difference or exception has been discovered (De Jong and Berg 2002). It is fascinating to observe how patients learn to expect this question, and not unusual for them to come to an appointment prepared for this query, having discussed it with others or contemplated it on their own. Table 7–1 shows solution-focused follow-up questions asking what is better.

TABLE 7–1.	Solution-focused follow-up questions: "What's better?"

- What's been better since I last saw you?
- What else has been better?
- Was this different?
- How was it different?
- Was it helpful?
- How was it helpful?
- How did you do it?
- Were things different between you and your VIPs because of this difference?
- How could I be most helpful for you so you can say this meeting has been beneficial and worthwhile for you?
- What are your best hopes for today's meeting?
- What is better between you and your VIPs?
- On a scale of 1–10, where 10 is you are satisfied with how things are between you and your VIPs and 1 is the opposite, where would you say things are now?
- Is this number going up or down?
- What makes it not lower?
- What else makes it not lower?
- What would it take to make it one point higher?
- On a scale of 1–10, where do you suppose your VIPs would rate how things are between you?
- On a scale of 1–10, how confident are you that you can continue to do what has been helpful for you?
- On a scale of 1–10, how confident do you think your VIPs are that you can continue doing what has been helpful for you?
- What would your VIPs say has been better?
- What else would your VIPs say has been better?
- On a scale of 1–10, how has school, home, work, family life, relationships been?

Asking patients how you can be most helpful to them so that they will be able to say it was beneficial and worthwhile for them to see you is an additional question that can be used during a follow-up session. Another version of this question is to ask what a patient's best hopes are for the session. These questions invite patients to take responsibility for what they want to accomplish from the meeting, while maintaining the focus on their goals and what is most important to them.

After asking what is better, detailing these freshly discovered assets, and eliciting best hopes for the meeting, it is helpful to ask scaling questions. Scaling questions can quickly evaluate a patient's function in myriad ways and from multiple perspectives. Scaling questions are remarkably constructive, especially when time afforded with patients is at a premium. Scaling questions invite patients to contemplate their subjective and personal experience in an unemotional and nonjudgmental way. A multitude of areas can be evaluated, such as work, school and home functioning, mood, relationship health, coping ability, medication effectiveness, motivation for change, confidence to attain goals, progress of treatment, and safety concerns, to name a few. Asking what makes the number not lower detects additional strengths. Asking what it would take to make the number go up by one point steers the conversation toward constructive and practical next steps that patients can take to attain their goals.

Case Illustration: Solution-Focused Follow-Up Session

Richard was a 13-year-old boy who was referred by his parents because of concerns about the diagnosis of attention-deficit/hyperactivity disorder (ADHD) and whether medications could be helpful for him. Review of his psychological testing, school evaluation, and parent reports substantiated the diagnosis of ADHD. Both parents reported they were diagnosed with ADHD and had benefited from medication treatment. During his initial evaluation, it was decided that a medication trial would be a reasonable option. The following session with Richard and his mother illustrates the subsequent session.

ANNE: What has been better since we last met?
I begin the conversation by asking what is better, immediately searching for positive differences.
RICHARD: I think I'm focusing better.
ANNE: What tells you that you are focusing better?
Asking people what "tells" them things are better conveys you believe they are thinking about this, subtly providing them a compliment.
RICHARD: I'm getting more of my work done and noticing more details.
ANNE: What else are you doing that tells you that you are focusing better?
A search for more details of this success continues.
RICHARD: I'm not getting into as many fights with my parents and I'm getting more of my work done.

ANNE: What else is better?

MOTHER: I notice he seems less frustrated and when I ask him to do things, he is retaining things better.

His mother chimes in with positive differences without being asked. If she hadn't done this, I would have directly asked her, in addition to Richard, what she notices is better with her son. It is important to obtain the patient's VIPs' perspectives of what is better.

ANNE: What else is he doing better?

MOTHER: He is doing things without being asked. He even washed the dog.

ANNE: Wow! That's a lot he is doing better. How do you think you have been able to do it?

A direct and indirect compliment are furnished.

RICHARD: I think the medications are helping me.

ANNE: That's great. Supposing 10 was the medication is helping like a magic pill and 1 the opposite, how much do you think the medication is helping you?

Scaling questions can quickly and easily assess medication effectiveness.

RICHARD: 7.

ANNE: That's great. What makes the number not lower?

RICHARD: I get my work done faster at school and my grades have really gone up.

ANNE: That's fantastic. You are working hard to help the medication work. What else makes it not lower?

I pair a compliment with a "what else" question gathering more details of this success.

RICHARD: I'm not fighting as much with my brother.

ANNE: What else makes it not lower?

RICHARD: My mom and I are getting along better.

A better relationship is an essential positive difference to amplify.

ANNE: Is this different that you are getting along better with your mother and brother?

RICHARD: Yes.

ANNE: How is it different?

RICHARD: My brother and I would fight all the time, and my mother would yell at me a lot because I wouldn't listen to her and would always argue with everything she said.

ANNE: Has that been helpful for you to get along better with your mother?

RICHARD: Yes.

ANNE: How has it been helpful?

RICHARD: We've been talking more and doing more things together.

ANNE: That's great. How are you doing this, getting along better?

RICHARD: I'm listening better and not arguing as much.

ANNE: How else are you able to get along better with your mother?

RICHARD: I'm also listening more and not arguing as much when she asks me to do things.

ANNE: That's fantastic! Suppose I had a scale from 1–10, where 10 is you are satisfied with how things are between you and your mother and 1 is the opposite, where would say things are?

Scaling questions quickly and easily assess the health of relationships.

RICHARD: 8.

ANNE: Is that number going up or down?

RICHARD: Up.

ANNE: And mom, how would you say things are between you and Richard on a scale of 1–10?

MOTHER: 8.

ANNE: Wow, that's a great number, and you both agree! What makes the number not lower for you?

MOTHER: I don't have to tell him to do things a hundred times before he will do them, and he's not arguing all the time when I ask him to do things. I don't get so frustrated.

ANNE: What else makes it not lower?

MOTHER: There is much less tension between us. We are getting along and having more time together. We played a board game the other night. We haven't done that in a while. I think it's because I got so frustrated with asking him to do things that I needed a break. Our relationship is definitely better.

This case illustrates a basic session in which things are better. Opportunities were taken to amplify positive differences and magnify both Richard's and his mother's accomplishments, increasing their self-efficacy. Medication effectiveness was evaluated and the patient's contribution to the medication's benefit highlighted. Attention was focused on the improvement of their relationship and the strengthening of the critical bond between Richard and his mother. Scaling questions were used to evaluate medication effectiveness, relationship health, and confidence that things could proceed in a positive direction. Although the session was only 30 minutes, a lot was accomplished in this brief amount of time.

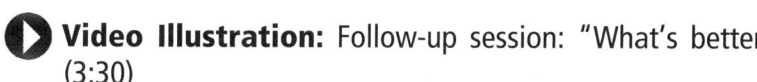 **Video Illustration:** Follow-up session: "What's better?" (3:30)

When Things Are Worse

There are times when patients cannot identify things that are better. When things are worse, it is still possible to remain solution focused. In these situations it is critical to provide enough emotional yes-set responses prior to embarking on questions. Asking patients what they have tried to do to handle these situations conveys they are working hard to solve their problems. Asking what they need in these situations assists them in discovering what they require to move forward. Asking them how they are coping with their problems reveals additional strengths and resources. Asking them where they get their strength compliments their hard work, fortitude, resilience, courage, and character, reinforcing their inner strength. Table 7–2 shows two key questions that can be asked when things are worse or in times of crisis.

TABLE 7–2.   **Questions that are useful when things are worse**

- What do you need?
- How are you coping?

What Do You Need?

The first question, "What do you need?", is a powerful solution-focused question that simultaneously conveys empathy and helps patients gain awareness of what they need. When patients are experiencing uncomfortable feelings such as anger, sadness, frustration, hopelessness, annoyance, anxiety, fear, panic, or worry, this provides a strong signal that they are encountering needs that are not being met. After providing an emotional yes-set response to how frustrating, sad, or annoying this must be "for them," it is then crucial to bridge this response with a solution-focused question. Notice that the question is not "What do you want?" Wants are different from needs. Needs are essential human requirements for survival. Asking patients what they need for themselves or from their VIPs helps to guide the conversation in a productive direction. Needs are often not explicitly stated, and when parents, children, spouses, and members of any form of dyad are in distress or conflict, helping them to articulate what they need from each other not only conveys empathy, but also directs the conversation constructively for everyone.

Asking patients what they need also connects to their emotional state. When patients are experiencing comfortable feelings, this generally indicates that what they are doing is in some way meeting their needs and is working for them. Uncomfortable feelings may indicate that patients are not having their needs met. Such feelings provide a red light where they can stop and think about what they need. Teaching patients about comfortable and uncomfortable feelings can help them learn the that both these types of feelings are beneficial for them in important ways, providing them a signal about whether what they are doing is meeting their needs. Mastering the ability to identify and tolerate uncomfortable feelings, connect these to unmet needs, and then act to get these needs met can be lifesaving. Not mastering these capabilities can have dangerous consequences. Uncomfortable feelings are red flags that there are unmet needs. Explaining to patients that feelings may be uncomfortable but are not dangerous can help them appreciate the function of uncomfortable feelings in getting what they need. In fact, when uncomfortable feelings and resulting unmet needs are ignored, this poses much greater risk. For example, many people who suffer from addiction use drugs to avoid painful and uncomfortable feelings; although in the immediate moment this may provide relief and what seems to them to be the only solution to their anguish, the consequences of ignoring the body's emotional pain can be devastating. People who have had early loss, trauma, attachment issues, and addiction often struggle with the skill of identifying and tolerating emotions, recognizing their unmet needs, and acting to meet these needs. They have good reason. They have frequently experienced agonizing emotional pain and not had their needs attended or responded to. They often have had experiences in which vocalizing their needs has been met with rejection, nonreaction, and inappropriate or inadequate responses. Learning to identify feelings, and to tolerate what at times may feel like intolerable emotions, requires enormous skill, courage, and faith that others will respond to these vocalized unmet needs. Ascertaining how these emotions relate to unmet needs, and then ultimately doing something about the situation so these needs can be met, is a very arduous endeavor and requires enormous skill to accomplish. Asking patients what they need helps them build these essential skills. It conveys empathy and signals that you appreciate they are having these feeling because a justifiable and pressing need of theirs is not being fulfilled. Asking them what they need conveys your belief in their ability to know what they need, if only asked.

Coping Questions

Coping questions are based on the appreciation of how painful and difficult life experiences are for many of the patients we see. When patients are faced with very challenging and painful life experiences, these questions can be particularly useful. Coping questions convey empathy with how difficult the situation is, while at the same time orienting the patient toward a small measure of success. The things a patient is doing to barely cope, however small they may be, are the very things he or she must do more of, one day at a time, to get through these challenging situations (De Jong and Berg 2002). Coping questions identify positive differences and exceptions to the patient's painful predicament (De Jong and Berg 1998; Fiske 2008). Patients are often unaware of the inner strengths and resources they have to cope with life unless specifically asked. These questions uncover critical resources that would otherwise go undetected. Coping questions are especially helpful in shifting the meaning of a patient's narrative from one of victimhood and self-blame to one of courage and strength to handle painful and challenging situations (Berg 1994). These shifts in meaning can help patients develop a sense of self-efficacy and reinforce a more hopeful view of their own capacity. Coping questions can be especially helpful in talking with parents who are overwhelmed, exhausted, and worried about their children. Taking the time to ask parents how they are coping and where they get their strength to continue often leads to answers that communicate how much they love their children and would do anything to help them.

These questions can liberate patients from their feelings of despair, inspiring a more optimistic perspective on their challenging predicament. The questions not only affirm what patients are doing to cope, but also communicate that the clinician is confident they can solve their own problems. Coping questions are especially useful when patients are in crisis (Fiske 2008). Pausing the conversation to explore positive decisions patients have made to cope and manage highlights the choices they are making, enhancing their sense of control. Noticing what positive actions patients take in crisis times is especially important to pursue—for example, noticing with patients how they made it to the appointment, found treatment for their child, didn't give up, got up and dressed in the morning, or made it to work in spite of their difficulties.

Case Illustration: Coping Questions

Megan was a 21-year-old girl pursuing a graduate degree in business. She was being treated for anxiety, obsessive-compulsive symptoms, and depression. She presented for a follow-up session in crisis: her boyfriend of more than two years had suddenly broken up with her. The following vignette illustrates how to incorporate coping questions in a crisis situation when things are worse.

ANNE: What's been better since we last met?

MEGAN: Nothing! Things are terrible. My boyfriend dumped me by text while I was visiting my family. It was horrible. On top of it, I have a terrible cold and just feel horrible.

ANNE: This must be so terrible for you.

It is important when patients are in significant distress to first supply "for you" emotional yes-set responses prior to asking questions.

MEGAN: (*She nods in agreement while crying.*)

ANNE: How have you been coping with all this?

MEGAN: Not well. I cried for three whole days and couldn't get out of bed. I just can't believe he broke up with me this way. The problem is that I still love him, but I feel like a fool if I take him back. I don't know whether this is truly it and the relationship has just run its course (*crying*).

ANNE: This must be very upsetting for you.

Because she is crying, more "for you" statements are required prior to asking a solution-focused question.

MEGAN: It was. I was so shocked and it was so upsetting. Now he's trying to get me back, but this is the second time he has done this and I don't think I should take him back. All my friends and family will think I'm a fool to take him back.

ANNE: This must be very difficult for you. How are you managing this?

I pair a "for you" response with a coping question.

MEGAN: I told him that I wouldn't see him until he got some help and therapy for at least a month.

Positive differences are frequently uncovered in response to a coping question.

ANNE: Have you asked him to do this before, or was this different?

This positive difference is then amplified.

MEGAN: This is different.

ANNE: How is it different?

MEGAN: Before, I kept letting things go. He would work all the time, but I would pay for everything. I'm sick of it. I need more from him.

ANNE: Was it helpful for you to ask him to get help?

MEGAN: I'm not sure he will even get it. I don't know.

ANNE: Supposing he would get help, what would you be doing differently?

This question can help clients gain control when they are basing their happiness on what others do. I incorporate her ideas about her boyfriend getting help, and then bridge this to a question about what she would be doing differently supposing he would get help. This redirects the conversation toward what she can do for herself, independently of him, and increases her sense of control.

MEGAN: I think I would have a better grip on my anxiety, although I think I am doing better with all this than I thought I would.

Another positive difference is revealed.

ANNE: What is better about how you are doing than you thought?

MEGAN: Well, the worst happened. He dumped me and I'm still standing.

ANNE: What do you mean by "standing"?

MEGAN: I'm sad, but fine.

ANNE: What are you doing that tells you that you are fine?

MEGAN: I'm going to class and meeting with my peers for our work.

More positive actions are discovered, and these can be complimented and amplified.

ANNE: Wow! That's great that you are able to do this in spite of how terrible you feel. What else tells you that you are fine?

MEGAN: I'm sleeping better after those initial few days, and getting up and working out.

ANNE: What else are you doing that tells you that you are fine?

MEGAN: I'm keeping myself busy, going grocery shopping and going to work. I made an appointment with my advisor about jobs and am seeing more friends.

ANNE: Is this different how you are coping with all of this?

MEGAN: Yes.

ANNE: How is it different?

MEGAN: I used to not do this and would just fall apart and call him back and go back to him.

ANNE: What are you doing instead of falling apart and calling him back?

I ask a "doing instead" question to redirect the conversation toward positive actions.

MEGAN: I'm spending more time with friends and focusing on my schoolwork and getting a job.

ANNE: Has this been helpful for you?

MEGAN: Yes.

ANNE: How has it been helpful for you?

MEGAN: I'm gaining confidence in myself.

ANNE: How are you able to do this, gain confidence in yourself?

MEGAN: I haven't been calling him and have been reaching out to my friends.

ANNE: Suppose 10 is you are satisfied with how you are coping and 1 is the opposite, where would you say you are now?

MEGAN: 5.

ANNE: What makes it not lower?

MEGAN: I'm getting to class, getting out of bed, and talking to my friends.

ANNE: What else makes it not lower?

MEGAN: I am gaining self-confidence and tolerating these feelings.

ANNE: What would it take to raise it by one point?

MEGAN: I think I just need more time away from him. I need to keep doing what I'm doing and not call him.

Coping questions and emotional yes-set responses are also important in the very difficult situations when parents are feeling so frustrated that they are unable to see anything positive in their children. When parents talk very negatively and have difficulties seeing positives in their children, despite a clinician's attempts to notice these with parents, it usually indicates that parents are exhausted and in need of more help and support for themselves. They need more compliments and "for you" statements for themselves prior to addressing their child's needs. This is often not what a clinician is inclined to do. It requires the clinician to suspend judgment and negative assumptions. Parents in these situations are easily frustrated and susceptible to feeling judged and blamed for being ineffectual and incompetent parents. This is the time to pay close attention in order to identify all the parental compliments you can find and to notice any and all parental positive differences within the conversation. Spending time building parental competencies, through the identification and amplification of positive differences, and uncovering hidden parental resources is imperative for effective treatment of children. Plenty of research demonstrates that in treatment of children, treating maternal depression has a large positive effect size (Pilowsky et al. 2008; Weissman et al. 2006; Wickramaratne et al. 2011). Blaming parents does little toward helping them help themselves or their children.

After parents have had enough time exploring their strengths, it is then important to begin to ask children what they most appreciate about their parents. A parent receiving a compliment from his or her own child is much more powerful than accolades from the treatment provider. Table 7–3 lists some questions to ask and responses to make when working with parents who find it difficult to identify strengths in their children.

TABLE 7–3.	Questions to ask parents who find it difficult to find strengths in their child

- This must be so difficult "for you."
- This must be so exhausting "for you."
- Where do you get your strength from?
- How have you managed to persevere?
- What has kept you from giving up on your child?
- How are you coping?
- How are you managing?
- What would your child say you do that is most helpful for him or her?
- What does the child see as your strengths as a parent?
- What do you need?
- What do you know about your child that tells the child he or she will succeed in life?
- Supposing 10 is you are satisfied with how you are coping with your child and 1 is the opposite, where would you say you are now?
- What makes it not lower?
- What else makes it not lower?
- What would it take to raise it by one point?

 Video Illustration: Coping questions (4:52)

Investigating for Details of Success: What Else, Who Else, How Else?

Effective solution building requires getting as many details as possible about successes and solutions (De Jong and Berg 2002). What else, who else, and how else are extremely powerful yet simple questions that amplify the details of success. These questions painstakingly leave no potential strength uncovered, and they are tremendously valuable conversational tools. Omitting asking "what else" questions carries great risk of missing undiagnosed crucial resources and potential solutions. These questions continue the pursuit of strengths until, figuratively speaking, no stone is left unturned. The "what else" questions (Table 7–4) can be adapted to many of the solution-focused questions. They are the metaphorical "language shovels" that dig for the details of success.

TABLE 7–4.   Questions that dig for details of success: what else?

- What else are you good at?
- What else do you enjoy?
- Who else is important in your life?
- What else do you appreciate about them?
- How else is it different?
- How else is it helpful?
- How else did you do it?
- What else is better?
- What else is better between you and your VIPs?
- What else makes the number not lower?
- What else would make it one point higher?
- What else would your VIPs say they appreciate about you?
- What else would your VIPs say is better?
- What else do you need?
- How else are you coping?
- What else do you know?
- What else do you know about your child that tells them they will succeed in life?
- What else will you be doing when your miracle day happens?
- What else will your VIPs notice you are doing on this miracle 10 day?

Case Illustration: What Else?

The following case illustrates how to use "what else" questions in a solu-tion-focused conversation. The case involves a 16-year-old girl, Nina, who is being treated for depression, addiction, and posttraumatic stress disorder. She was being treated in an inpatient setting after making suicidal threats. This vignette begins when the clinician asks about her VIPs. Notice how the "what else" questions uncover tremendous resources and direct the conversation toward the patient's goals. I reiterate these questions below to illustrate how often and how powerfully they can be asked.

ANNE: I am wondering, who are the most important people in your life?
NINA: My family.
ANNE: Who is most important in your family?
NINA: My mother, father, and grandmother.
ANNE: Who else is important in your life?
NINA: My niece and my sister.
ANNE: Who else is most important in your life?
NINA: My stepfather. He has been there more than my real father.

ANNE: Who else?

NINA: I don't know. That's it.

This response indicates it is time to move forward with other questions.

ANNE: You have a lot of people you care about. What do you appreciate most about your mother?

I provide a direct compliment prior to moving forward with questions.

NINA: She doesn't give up on me. No matter how bad it got.

ANNE: What else do you appreciate about her?

NINA: She cares about me.

ANNE: How do you know she cares?

NINA: She does whatever it takes to get me the help I need.

ANNE: How else do you know she cares?

NINA: She comes and visits me. It takes almost two hours to get here, but she always is here.

I continue asking what else she appreciates about her mother until she can no longer identify things. I then begin to ask her what she appreciates about her grandmother.

ANNE: What do you appreciate most about your grandmother?

NINA: She is always there for me. She's like a second mother to me.

ANNE: What do you mean second mother?

NINA: I lived with her. She made me go to school.

ANNE: Wow! What else do you appreciate about her?

I now do the same line of questioning with another VIP she has identified.

NINA: She made me get help. She supported my mother, too.

ANNE: What else do you appreciate about her?

I continue to ask what else she appreciates about her grandmother until she cannot identify anything further. I then proceed to ask what she appreciates most about the other important people in her life: her sister, stepfather, and niece. Each time, I pursue what else she appreciates about each of them until nothing further is revealed. In this way, I am highlighting her relationship strengths. These supports will be critical for her recovery. The conversation continues and she brings up painful emotions she has experienced as she comes to terms with how her addiction has hurt her family. The following is an excerpt from this portion of the session, illustrating more uses for the "what else" question.

ANNE: This must be very difficult for you to think about how you hurt your mother and grandmother. How have you coped with this?

I begin by providing her a "for you" response, followed by a coping question.

NINA: They [mother and grandmother] don't believe or trust me. I know I have hurt them. I even made my grandmother cry. That really bothered me. I just need to be honest with them. I want to tell her I lost her ring here. I know she won't believe me. She'll think I sold it. But I just need to tell her this.

She discloses very sensitive information. This is not unusual when patients are feeling listened to and understood.

ANNE: I can see how much you care about your mother and grandmother. It takes a lot of courage to be able to talk about difficult things like this. Is this something you have always been good at?
I explore whether her ability to talk about difficult things may be a positive difference.
NINA: I guess so. Some people would call it stubbornness.
ANNE: What do mean by stubbornness?
NINA: Doing what I want, whenever I want. I would never take *no* without arguing. But now I am trying to tell the truth and be honest, and they don't trust me.
ANNE: That must be difficult for you that they don't trust you. Is it different that you are now trying to tell the truth and be honest?
Another potential difference has been revealed, honesty.
NINA: Yes. I would never do that when I was using.
ANNE: Has it been helpful for you?
NINA: Yes.
ANNE: How has it been helpful?
NINA: I am slowly beginning to regain their trust.
ANNE: How else has it been helpful to be honest with them?
NINA: Our relationship is getting better. We're having better phone calls.
ANNE: How are you able to do this?
NINA: I'm learning a lot of things here.
ANNE: All that you are learning is so impressive. I can tell how hard you are working. What else have you been learning?
NINA: I'm learning how to do my chores and behave.
ANNE: What else are you learning?
NINA: I'm learning to not swear.
ANNE: What are you doing instead of swearing?
NINA: I'm learning to watch my tone.
ANNE: What else are you learning?
NINA: I'm learning to follow rules.
ANNE: Wow! That's a lot you are learning. It's not easy following all the rules they have here. How are you managing to learn all this?

This excerpt illustrates the power of "what else." Persisting in asking what else, who else, and how else questions is a powerful conversational tool that assists in leaving no potential strength undiscovered.

Questions That Amplify Ambivalence

Learning how to amplify ambivalence with patients is an essential skill in learning how to become solution focused. Amplifying ambivalence is an important step toward increasing motivation to change (Miller and Rollnick 2002). Ambivalence is normal for all people and an important feature in helping people articulate goals and choices in their life. All people are ambivalent about the many choices they make. Should you eat that second piece of cake? Should you get up in the morning and exercise? Should you watch TV or read a book? Asking how seemingly unhelpful behaviors are helpful and eliciting a client's "good reason" for the chosen behaviors amplifies ambivalence.

Amplifying ambivalence is especially important when patients are doing things that are harmful to themselves or to others, have no desire to seek treatment, are in denial about their need for help, or are externally motivated. In these situations, it is helpful to remember that unless the contrary is proven, we can assume people choose to act in ways that are in some way beneficial for them. Maintaining this assumption can be challenging, especially when patients are engaging in harmful behaviors. How can a clinician affirm patients in these circumstances, while also attending to safety and protective issues? Staying calm and putting your own assumptions on the back burner can be difficult. In these situations, it can be tempting to fall into the trap of telling people what to do or giving unsolicited advice. Asking questions that invite patients to help explain their choice of behaviors, even if the behaviors are harmful, conveys respect and a desire to understand without judgment.

In working to amplify ambivalence, it is essential to know who a patient's VIPs are and what those people most appreciate about the patient, as well as to discover his or her strengths and talents. After this discussion, the solution-focused clinician begins to amplify ambivalence by first asking how a harmful behavior is helpful for the patient. Beginning with how a behavior is helpful for the patient maintains agreement within the conversation. When the clinician asks how drugs are helpful, and how else they are helpful, and how else they are helpful, patients often eventually say they are not helpful. This indicates that it is then time to ask how these behaviors are unhelpful. Asking how drugs are helpful, how hitting their child is helpful, how cutting themselves or thinking about suicide is helpful, fosters a desire to know and understand more and invites patients to explain their reasoning in an affirming way. It is not unusual for patients to appear perplexed by these questions. Explaining that their behaviors must in some way be helpful for them, or they would not continue them, maintains the nonassuming stance while concomitantly placing the responsibility for the choices they are making onto them. This can gently amplify their ambivalence. It also often opens up the dialog in an honest way as patients see the clinician striving to understand their perspective in an accepting and nonjudgmental fashion. When a patient identifies how drugs help them relax and avoid emotional pain, a discussion can then proceed about what other things they have tried to do to relax or cope with their emotional pain. If patients state their behaviors are not helpful, asking what they could "do instead" redirects the conversation toward their goals, increasing their motivation to change. This order of questioning, beginning with the helpful aspects of harmful behaviors, is critical. This order of inquiry amplifies ambivalence while simultaneously building the therapeutic alliance.

There are times when patients cannot identify any unhelpful aspects of their harmful behaviors. If this happens, it is essential to ask how helpful or unhelpful their VIPs would rate these behaviors to be. Often, patients reply that VIPs would rate their behaviors as unhelpful, and articulating this can help patients notice the effect of their behaviors on those most important to them, increasing their motivation to change.

Scaling questions are very useful in amplifying ambivalence. Asking how helpful or unhelpful behaviors are from 1–10, from both patients' and their VIPs' perspective, assesses motivation to change while amplifying ambivalence and directing the conversation toward solutions.

When patients are engaging in harmful behaviors, you can also ask what Insoo Kim Berg called the "good reason" question (De Jong and Berg 2002). Asking patients their good reason for their harmful behaviors invites them to explain how these actions are beneficial for them, while maintaining the clinician's nonjudgmental and agreeable stance. It respectfully communicates to patients that they are the experts on the reasons for their behaviors, and it conveys their responsibility and choice in the actions they are taking.

When patients are asked their good reasons for using drugs, they often say drugs relieve their emotional pain and help them escape from the pain of their reality, cope with traumatic experiences, numb uncomfortable feelings, make friends, feel happy, and have fun. Asking the "good reason" question reorients the conversation toward appreciating how patients are coping, and it can then lead the conversation toward other ways they have coped or would like to cope in these difficult life circumstances. Asking the "good reason" question is quite different from asking "why" a patient is engaging in a harmful behavior. "Why" questions often generate a defensive position and decrease engagement and agreement within the conversation, none of which promotes a collaborative dialog that generates solutions. There are specific questions that can be used to amplify ambivalence (Table 7–5).

Case Illustration: Amplifying Ambivalence in a Self-Harming Adolescent

Emily was a 16-year-old girl being treated for addiction at a drug rehabilitation center. Her drugs of choice were alcohol, cannabis, prescription opioids, and nicotine. Her probation officer mandated her into treatment after she failed several drug tests. Emily had a long history of sexual abuse by her father. She was living with her mother prior to her admission, and recently her mother was diagnosed with a relapse of breast cancer. Emily had been a caretaker for her family for many years. Her mother did not want her to come

TABLE 7–5.   Questions that amplify ambivalence

- Is _____ [insert harmful behavior] helpful for you?
- How is it helpful for you?
- How else is it helpful for you?
- Supposing 10 is this behavior is very helpful for you and 1 is the opposite, how helpful do you think the behavior is for you?
- How helpful would your VIPs rate this behavior for you from 1–10?
- How unhelpful would your VIPs rate this behavior from 1–10?
- You must have a good reason to _____ [insert harmful behaviors]?
- What else is your good reason?

into treatment because of her own need to have Emily help at home. I was asked to evaluate her because she was cutting herself and staff were concerned about her safety. The following is an excerpt from this conversation.

ANNE: What's been better since I last saw you?

I begin the conversation by asking what's better. This immediately moves the conversation toward identification of positive differences. It may feel counterintuitive to begin the conversation with her strengths, given the level of safety concerns, but this is an essential conversational step. More conversational deposits and "anesthesia" are required for the difficult questions ahead. Omitting this step runs the risk of missing crucial resources she will need to cope.

EMILY: I am considering college. They had a volunteer speaker from a college that came here and spoke to us about options available when you go to college.

A potential positive difference is revealed. Thinking about college is forward thinking and is important to amplify.

ANNE: Is this different that you are considering the option of college for yourself?

EMILY: Yes.

ANNE: How is it different that you are considering college as an option?

EMILY: I used to think I was never going to go to college. My eyes were closed to possibilities.

ANNE: Is this helpful for you to open your eyes to this possibility?

I incorporate "opening" her eyes, linguistically underscoring possibility.

EMILY: Yes.

ANNE: How is it helpful for you to open your eyes to this possibility?

EMILY: I didn't have expectations for myself. The staff has helped me open my eyes to more possibilities.

ANNE: Wow! How did you do this, open your eyes to these possibilities for yourself?

EMILY: I think part of it is that I am sober and thinking clearly. It sounds kind of silly, but I'm seeing that with effort, I can maybe change something in the world.

Critical resources (positive differences) that may have been left undetected are discovered and can now be amplified.

ANNE: That doesn't sound silly at all. Is this different for you to see how you may be able to change things in the world?

EMILY: Yes.

ANNE: How is it different that you are seeing how you may be able to change things in the world?

EMILY: I would never think about myself. I really want to figure myself out.

Another positive difference is discovered.

ANNE: Has this been helpful for you to think more about yourself?

EMILY: Yes.

ANNE: How has it been helpful to think more about yourself and try to figure yourself out?

EMILY: I want to be able to better myself and do positive things in my life. I never thought I would be able to do that.

ANNE: I am impressed with all the hard work you are doing. How you are considering new options for yourself, opening your eyes to new possibilities, thinking clearly now that you are sober, seeing the positive things in your life, including how you could make changes in the world, and working so hard to figure yourself out and better yourself. This is hard and very impressive work you are doing here. I hope you will continue to do more of this impressive work. The staff had asked me to see you today because they are worried about you. Would it be OK if I change the subject a bit?

In working with patients who are engaging in harmful behaviors, it is critical to provide them with as many realistic and genuine compliments as possible prior to asking solution-focused questions. Only after positive differences have been identified, amplified, and then summarized in a list of compliments is it time to more directly address the staff's concerns. I respectfully give the patient a heads-up about a question that is different from the current direction of the conversation. I intentionally phrase the question to integrate what the staff "are worried about," conveying their concern.

EMILY: It's OK.

ANNE: Did you know that staff was worried about you?

I ask if she knew that the staff members were worried, conveying their concern.

EMILY: No (*pause*). I guess (*holding her face in her hands*). I don't want to talk about that.

I chose to wait a moment, and she did acknowledge the staff concern.

ANNE: Of course, that makes sense that this is very difficult for you to talk about. Do you know what the staff are worried about that they thought it might be a good idea to see me?

I bridge a "for you" response with a question exploring her perception of the staff concerns, conveying her knowledge and expertise.

EMILY: That I have been cutting.

ANNE: You are not alone with this. Many clients here have struggled with cutting. You must have a good reason to cut yourself?

I reassure her that she is not unusual, and then bridge this normalizing response with the "good reason" question.

EMILY: It helps me to forget about all my problems.

ANNE: How else is it helpful for you to cut yourself?
> *When amplifying ambivalence, it is important to begin with how harmful behaviors are in some way beneficial for them.*

EMILY: I can't stand the emotional pain. I just don't know how to get rid of it. It seems easier to cut myself.

ANNE: This must be so difficult for you. I can tell how hard you are working to feel better. How does cutting help you cope with your emotional pain?
> *I bridge a "for you" response and a compliment with a coping question.*

EMILY: I am able to focus on physical pain, and this is easier to deal with. I can clean it, put a Band-Aid on it, and do something to take care of it. I can't do that with my emotional pain.

ANNE: Of course, that makes sense. Learning how to deal with emotional pain is very difficult. How else is cutting helpful for you?
> *I provide a general yes-set response and a normalizing response with a "how is this helpful" question, continuing to amplify her ambivalence.*

EMILY: It's a way I can deal with my anger. I have a real problem with anger.

ANNE: Supposing 10 is cutting yourself is very helpful for you and 1 is the opposite, how helpful would you say it is for you now?
> *Scaling questions further amplify her ambivalence by exploring her perception of how helpful or unhelpful these behaviors are for her.*

EMILY: 4.

ANNE: And how unhelpful would you say it is?

EMILY: 7.

ANNE: How is cutting yourself unhelpful for you?

EMILY: I have all these scars and it causes me to end up in places like this.

ANNE: How else is cutting yourself unhelpful for you?

EMILY: I don't end up earning a pass and then can't see my family. My mom gets upset with me, too.

ANNE: How helpful do you think your mother would say cutting is for you?
> *Scaling her VIP's perception of helpfulness further amplifies ambivalence.*

EMILY: 0.

ANNE: And how unhelpful do you think she would say it is?

EMILY: 10!

This case illustrates how to ask questions that amplify ambivalence. These questions can be used with any types of behaviors that are harmful, such as substance abuse, self-harming behaviors, thoughts of suicide, people staying in domestically violent relationships, parents hitting their children, or children getting into trouble at school.

LEARNING EXERCISE: PRACTICING QUESTIONS

Have people break into groups of three, one person acting as a clinician, one person as a patient, and one person as an observer. Have the members of the group take turns practicing working with a patient who is engaging in harmful behaviors by asking questions that amplify ambivalence. Also have the members practice questions used in follow-up sessions, both when things are better and when things are worse. Continue to practice integrating "for you" statements, yes-set responses, compliments, and use of a patient's exact words, working to gain skill in creating shared dialects within conversations. Have the observer comment on what he or she noticed were particularly helpful questions that promoted solutions within the conversation.

By this time, you are well on your way to becoming a solution-focused clinician. Structuring an interview in a solution-focused format often will elicit a wealth of needed information. However, there is the reality that as clinicians, we work in a world that also requires us to gather necessary information that may have not been gathered by the questions and techniques described thus far. The following chapter will present a method for conducting a solution-focused review of systems in order to address this need.

KEY POINTS

- A solution-focused follow-up session begins by asking "What's better?"

- Other possible follow-up questions include "What are your best hopes for the session today?" and "How could I be most helpful for you today?"

- Scaling questions can evaluate a patient's function in myriad ways from multiple perspectives and are quick and simple to ask in follow-up sessions.

- When things are worse, it is essential to pair enough "for you" responses and compliments with coping questions and "What do you need" questions.

- Asking patients what they need guides the conversation toward solutions while at the same time conveying empathy.

- Coping questions convey empathy while at the same time orienting the patient toward a small measure of success.

- Coping questions help to shift the patient narrative from one of victimhood and self-blame to one of courage and strength to handle life's challenging situations.

- "What else," "who else," and "how else" questions are the metaphorical "language shovels" that dig for and amplify a patient's successes.

- A solution-focused clinician amplifies ambivalence by first exploring how harmful behaviors are helpful for patients and eliciting their "good reason" for choosing these behaviors.

- "Why" questions often generate defensiveness on the part of patients, weakening the therapeutic alliance.

References

Berg IK: Family Based Services: A Solution-Focused Approach. New York, WW Norton, 1994

De Jong P, Berg IK: Interviewing for Solutions. Belmont, CA, Brooks/Cole, 1998

De Jong P, Berg IK: Interviewing for Solutions, 2nd Edition. Pacific Grove, CA, Brooks/Cole, 2002

Fiske H: Hope in Action: Solution-Focused Conversations About Suicide. New York, Routledge/Taylor & Francis Group, 2008

Miller WR, Rollnick S: Motivational Interviewing: Preparing People for Change. New York, Guilford, 2002

Pilowsky DJ, Wickramaratne P, Talati A, et al: Children of depressed mothers 1 year after the initiation of maternal treatment: findings from the STAR*D-Child Study. Am J Psychiatry 165:1136–1147, 2008

Weissman MM, Pilowsky DJ, Wickramaratne PJ, et al: Remissions in maternal depression and child psychopathology: a STAR*D-child report. JAMA 295:1389–1398, 2006

Wickramaratne P, Gameroff MJ, Pilowsky DJ, et al: Children of depressed mothers 1 year after remission of maternal depression: findings from the STAR*D-Child study. Am J Psychiatry 168:593–602, 2011

CHAPTER 8

Solution-Focused Assessment

Completing a psychiatric and clinical evaluation is a highly skilled endeavor requiring expertise in many areas, including that of obtaining the necessary information to treat patients most effectively (Dulcan 2010; Hales and Yudofsky 2003). One question that often arises in learning solution-focused therapy is how to balance maintaining a solution-focused conversation with the need to obtain required diagnostic information. All fields of medicine have required standards of care and best practices (Norcross et al. 2008; Stout and Hayes 2005). These not only provide guidance for clinicians in the field, but also are the benchmarks to which professionals are held should the unexpected happen and a patient have a poor outcome. A good clinician takes these standards to heart regardless of the theoretical model employed. Each theoretical approach may have a different focus of assessment and treatment, but regardless of model, there are common domains that measure treatment effectiveness. These areas include quality of life, patient functioning in multiple domains, and whether the patient and his or her VIPs (very important people) view their problem as solved. These criteria determine whether treatment has been successful. In this way, the solution-focused model of treatment shares the identified problem and outcome criteria of other treatment models. The difference is how the solution-focused clinician guides the conversation toward these discharge criteria. Let's use the analogy of a snowball at the top of a mountain. If you begin with a small snowball at the top of the mountain and proceed to build this snowball by asking solution-focused questions, the end result at the bottom of the mountain, the end of the conversation, will be a huge snowball with many identified solutions. If you begin with the same snowball but instead ask many problem-focused questions, the end result will be a huge snowball expounding the details of many problems.

Solution-Focused Review of Systems

This chapter will focus on how to perform a solution-focused review of systems. Performing a review of systems is important in conducting clinical evaluations so that important information is not missed (American Psychiatric Association 2006). Areas covered in a review of systems may include substance use, trauma, suicide, safety, mood, anxiety, prior psychiatric treatment, family history, developmental issues, and information required to meet agency and clinic standards. A solution-focused review of systems collects this required information while expanding the strength-based narrative.

The solution-focused therapy model does not presume that the solution to patients' problems is necessarily linked to the cause of their problems. How can a solution-focused therapist maintain a solution-focused conversation while gathering the required diagnostic information that is focused on the detection and elaboration of problems? How can both be accomplished? As can be seen from the previous chapters and case illustrations, becoming a solution-focused therapist does not mean you are inattentive to patients' problems. Solution-focused therapists are acutely aware of patients' problems, but these problems are appreciated from within a narrative of patient strength, through the use of carefully constructed solution-focused questions. Patients' problems are contextualized and viewed through a competency-based lens, creating a narrative based on capabilities and successes rather than diagnosis and pathology.

A solution-focused clinician is well aware of potential clinical issues, such as depression, anxiety, attention-deficit/hyperactivity disorder (ADHD), trauma, disrupted attachment, substance abuse, medication use, suicide, and risk of self-harm, and has the same goals as other clinicians: to help patients solve their problems, resulting in a successful treatment outcome. The difference is how a solution-focused therapist evaluates these issues employing the lens of solution-focused questions and techniques. In fact, when solution-focused techniques are practiced well, often a more honest and detailed view of the problem arises.

Clinicians are frequently required to function in many roles. These may include performing individual therapy, family therapy, medication consultation, crisis management, safety evaluations, advocacy, parent management training, school consultation, consultations to other medical providers, and care coordination, to name a few. All of these responsibilities require excellent assessment skills. Solution-focused assessment involves asking different questions, and in a different order, than those asked in problem-focused assessments. For example, when a child presents with anger issues, a solution-focused therapist would start in the same way as discussed in previous chapters, exploring strengths, VIPs, and best hopes for treatment. The clinician might ask children with these issues what they do to calm down, how they manage frustration, what has stopped them from hitting another child a second or third time, their "good reason" for their anger, their best hopes when they are able to manage their frustration, and how satisfied they are in their ability to calm down on a scale of 1–10.

The solution-focused review of systems is performed after completion of the initial solution-focused interview that includes the identification of strengths, VIPs, best hopes for treatment, miracle question, and scaling questions. It is helpful to prepare patients for the change in the conversational direction prior to carrying out the review of systems. Asking patients whether it would be OK to put on "a doctor hat" and ask more "doctor-type medical questions," so that important information is not missed, respectfully accomplishes this conversational transition. Patients are generally more than willing to accommodate this request, especially after participating in the preceding solution-focused conversation. This effectively separates the interview into two sections, the solution-focused interview and the solution-focused review of systems.

The solution-focused review of systems includes assessing domains of mood, relationships, safety, ADHD, anxiety, trauma, eating disorders, attachment, social skills, substance abuse, past psychiatric history, family history, and medical issues. Learning solution-focused therapy requires being on constant alert for positive differences. Grouping positive differences into diagnostic categories can be helpful to learn, much like learning diagnostic symptom categories. Table 8–1 provides a few examples.

Solution-Focused Mood Assessment

Anhedonia, the lack of enjoyment in life, is a critical area to evaluate in assessing mood (Hersen 2004). Anhedonia has already been assessed by the very first questions asked in a solution-focused interview, when patients are asked what they are good at and enjoy. When patients are unable to identify anything they are good at or enjoy, this signals that they may be experiencing anhedonia. Asking patients about their sleep and appetite are neutral questions often perceived as nurturing and caring, and these are important areas to evaluate when assessing mood. Scaling questions can easily assess mood and are often comfortably answered by patients. Asking patients how they would rate their mood from 1–10, where 10 is they are satisfied with how they are feeling and 1 is the opposite, obtains a subjective assessment of a patient's mood. Asking what makes the number not lower amplifies resources, hope, coping strategies, and plans for the future. When patients rate their mood as a 1 or even a negative number, a solution-focused con-

TABLE 8–1.	Positive differences grouped according to diagnostic categories

- **Mood:** Identifying things one is good at and enjoys, feeling happy, experiencing more energy, staying calm in the face of conflict, experiencing pleasure, doing fun things, seeking social interaction, thinking positively, asserting one's needs, asking for help, accepting help, displaying future orientation, imagining goals, concentrating and focusing, having reasons for living

- **ADHD:** Stopping and thinking things through before acting, focusing, paying attention, planning, getting work done, remaining calm physically, waiting, organizing homework, remembering homework

- **Anxiety:** Approaching situations that are anxiety provoking, utilizing relaxation skills, experiencing a calm and relaxed state in mind and body

- **Substance abuse:** Cutting down on use, gaining sober time no matter how short-lived, getting a sponsor, going to meetings, thinking clearly, being honest, acting responsibly, managing cravings, thinking things through

versation can still be maintained by asking how they have coped in the face of these difficulties, where they get their strength from, and how they managed to come to the appointment despite the challenges they face. When patients rate their number as very low, it also becomes a red flag for the clinician to evaluate a patient's safety.

Providing education is an important intervention for all clinicians, and diagnosing depression can be helpful when symptoms are externalized as part of the disease instead of an inherent flaw of the patient. Externalizing the disease of depression can also help to minimize blame and make it easier for patients, children, and their parents and other VIPs to work together toward a common goal of fighting this problem.

Asking whether parents or other family members have suffered from depression, how they have coped with these difficulties, and what things they have tried to do to help yields important family history information while maintaining an empathic narrative built around strength and resilience. A solution-focused therapist does not directly ask if anyone in the family has been "diagnosed with" depression, but instead inquires if anyone has "suffered" from or has "coped" with depression. Choosing the word "suffer" conveys empathy, which promotes engagement while gathering the necessary family history. Choosing the work "coped" communicates they have managed despite the challenges. Asking what has been most helpful for family members who have coped with depression uncovers potential valuable treatment options that may be crucial when treating your patient. All of these questions provide opportunities to compliment patients on their strengths and coping skills, inviting them to become more aware of how they are managing in the face of difficult life circumstances.

 Video Illustration: Mood assessment (4:15)

Solution-Focused Assessment of Relationship Health

The health of important relationships in a patient's life is a crucial domain to evaluate in a solution-focused review of systems. Much like vital signs in a medical evaluation, relationship health is imperative to assess in a solution-focused evaluation. Asking patients how things are "between" them and their VIPs from 1–10 can quickly assess the health of important relationships in their life. Asking what makes the number not lower highlights what is working in the relationship and provides opportunities to amplify these strengths. Asking what it will take to raise the number by one point facilitates the next steps they need to take to improve their relationship. Scaling the strength of relationships can be done with parents, children, spouses, siblings, or any identified VIPs.

Scaling relationship health is especially important in working with parents and children. Children learn how to regulate their emotions first and foremost through the interaction with their parents or other primary caretakers. In assessing relationship health in children, it is imperative to assess how parents regulate their own emotions and stay calm in the face of conflict and challenging situations. When parents are able to remain calm, empathize with their children, and provide emotional yes-set responses, all while maintaining limits, the children learn how to regulate their emotions.

Parents' mood can significantly affect the mood and behaviors of their children (Coiro et al. 2012; Wickramaratne et al. 2011). Providing education to parents on their critical role in modeling and teaching emotional regulation skills is therefore time well spent. When a parent is required to set a limit on his or her child and the child becomes angry or acts out, the parent needs to remain calm while maintaining this boundary. This requires great skill on the part of parents, many of whom have not had these learning opportunities. Asking parents how well they are able to remain calm, follow through on limits, and validate their child's experiences from 1–10 assesses these important parental skills in a nonjudgmental way and provides another measurement of relationship health. These questions can also be used in working with couples, siblings, or people in other types of relationships.

Listening for and amplifying parents' positive emotional regulation skills, such as staying calm while maintaining a limit on a child, offers opportunities to provide direct and indirect compliments. Normalizing with parents how difficult this skill is for many people, and asking how they learned to modulate their own emotions, provides empathy while uncovering additional strengths. It is helpful to explain to parents that their ability to remain calm often results in a stronger bond between parent and child and provides learning opportunities for the child to manage his or her own emotions. Remaining calm prevents a cycle in which both the child's and the parent's emotions escalate. Scaling from 1–10 how well parents can remain calm when setting limits or how they would rate their ability to manage their child's emotional challenges can further evaluate relationship health. Table 8–2 lists solution-focused questions that assess relationship health.

TABLE 8–2.	Solution-focused questions to evaluate relationship health with children and other VIPs

- How would you rate things "between" you and your VIPs from 1–10, where 10 is you are satisfied with your relationship and 1 is the opposite?
- How do you suppose your VIPs would rate things "between" the two of you on a scale of 1–10?
- What makes the number not lower?
- What else makes it not lower?
- What would make it one point higher?
- How well are you able to remain calm from 1–10 when setting a limit with your child?
- How well are you able to follow through on limits with your child from 1–10, where 10 is you are satisfied and 1 is the opposite?
- What makes the number not lower?
- What would make it one point higher?
- Where do you suppose your child, or other VIPs, would rate your ability to remain calm from 1–10?

Solution-Focused Assessment of Anger

When patients present with anger problems, the following questions can be asked during a solution-focused review of systems. Asking patients how they calm down and manage frustration conveys that they possess the skills to do so. When children have problems with physical aggression, asking their "good reason" for aggressive behavior such as hitting others, whether aggression is helpful for them, how they stop hitting others, and what stopped them from hitting others a second or third time addresses issues of anger while uncovering positive differences and solutions to these difficulties. Asking what patients have tried to do to cope with these difficulties provides opportunities to compliment them on how hard they have already been working to solve their problems.

In working with patients who struggle with aggression, it is useful to remember that such problems do not happen all the time. It is important to pause to explore and amplify positive differences that are notable when the problem is less severe or is not happening. Was it different during the times when they were able to stay out of trouble? Was it helpful for them to stay out of trouble? How was it helpful? How did they do it? Were things different between them and their VIPs when they were able to stay out of trouble? What did their VIPs notice they are doing differently when they are able to stay out of trouble and remain calm? When there have been fights, how have they stopped? What stopped them from hitting someone a second or third time? Was it different when they didn't get into a fight and were able to stay calm? How confident are they that they will stay out of trouble and remain calm from 1–10? What makes it not lower, and what would make it one point higher? How confidently would their VIPs rate their ability to stay out of trouble or calm down from 1–10? Table 8–3 lists solution-focused questions that can be helpful to ask patients with anger issues.

Solution-Focused Assessment of Safety

Inquiring about suicidal and self-harming behaviors is important in evaluating safety issues (Simon and Hales 2006). Preparing patients for questions that evaluate safety by explaining that these are routinely asked helps to normalize their struggles, aiding them in feeling less alone.

Framing questions about safety in the context of "pain" and "good reason" conveys empathy with the intense suffering patients may be experiencing. It conveys that they have a reason for thinking about suicide as an option: to rid themselves of their intense agony. When patients have contemplated suicide and not followed through, it is important to ask what stopped them from acting on these thoughts. Patients usually respond by talking about important people and relationships in their life such as their children, parents, spouse, and even pets. This provides opportunities to explore more about the connections and relationships that are of great importance to them. These VIP relationships are generally the ones that will prevent patients from acting in these destructive ways. Uncovering these relationships and amplifying the positive aspects of a patient's VIPs can be life saving.

Asking patients their reasons for living guides the conversation toward their hopes, goals, and future dreams (Fiske 2008). Scaling their reasons for

TABLE 8–3.	Solution-focused questions that can be helpful to ask patients with anger issues

- On a scale of 1–10, where 10 is you are able to calm down and 1 is the opposite, where would you rate things?
- On a scale of 1–10, where 10 is you are able to stay out of trouble and 1 is the opposite, where would you say you are now?
- Where would your VIPs rate your ability to stay out of trouble and calm down from 1–10?
- You must have a good reason for getting so angry?
- Has it been helpful for you to get angry?
- What have you tried to do to calm down?
- What else have you tried to do to calm down?
- What stopped you from hitting someone a second time?
- How did you stop hitting the person a second time?
- How have you managed to calm down?
- How confident are you on a scale of 1–10 that you can calm down and manage your anger?
- How confident are your VIPs that you can manage your anger on a scale of 1–10?
- What makes the number not lower?
- What else makes it not lower?
- What would make it one point higher?

living from 1–10, where 10 is they are satisfied with their reasons for living and 1 is the opposite, can uncover thoughts about their hopes, aspirations, and goals for the future. As discussed in the previous chapters, starting with questions about how harmful behaviors are helpful amplifies ambivalence and frequently leads patients to realize these behaviors are not useful for them. These questions can then be followed up with scaling questions about how helpful or unhelpful they and their VIPs perceive these harmful actions to be and what they could do instead.

Solution-focused questions are valuable in safety planning and risk assessment. Scaling questions can collaboratively concretize a safety plan in detailed behavioral ways (Fiske 2008). What would tell patients they are confident, at a 10, that they can keep themselves safe? What would they be doing at a 10? What else would they be doing? How confident are they from 1–10 that they can keep themselves safe? How confidently would they predict their VIPs would rate their ability to keep themselves safe on a scale from 1–10? What would make the number not lower? What else would make it not lower? What would make it one point higher? At what number would they require a higher level of care? At what number would their VIPs say they require a higher level of care? How confident are their VIPs on a scale from 1–10 that they can remain safe? How confident from 1–10 are their VIPs that they can do the necessary things to help keep the patient safe?

Asking these questions collaboratively develops a concrete safety plan with the patient and his or her VIPs. Writing down the details of this plan on an index card and giving it to the patient solidifies this plan, which can then be documented in the patient record. Additional phone numbers can also be added to this index card, including emergency mental health numbers, hotline numbers, phone numbers of VIPs, and any other resources or ideas that were discussed that were determined to be of help for the patient.

When a patient requires a higher level of care, the following questions can help to sustain a solution-focused conversation that encourages both patients and their VIPs to be involved in this difficult decision, while conferring a sense of control and responsibility. What are the patient's best hopes for hospitalization? What are the patient's VIP's best hopes for the hospitalization? How is the patient hoping the hospitalization will be helpful? What will tell the patient that he or she is ready to leave the hospital and has learned the necessary skills to keep safe? What will tell the patient's VIPs that they have learned the necessary skills to help the patient?

For clinicians who are referring a patient for hospitalization, it is helpful to contact the admitting hospital and think about what your best hopes are for the patient's hospitalization and communicate this to the treatment team who is caring for your patient. How are you, as the clinician, hoping the hospitalization would be helpful for your patient? What are you hoping to get help with from the treatment team who is caring for your patient? Communicating this to the treatment team and expressing appreciation for their help in the care of your patient promotes a collaborative relationship with the treatment team. Table 8–4 lists solution-focused questions that evaluate safety issues.

Video Illustration: Safety assessment (4:13)

Case Illustration: Solution-Focused Safety Assessment

Christine was a 45-year-old grandmother who had been receiving treatment for posttraumatic stress disorder, depression, and substance abuse. She had suffered from years of trauma, and recently her son was murdered. She experienced suicidal episodes, especially around the anniversary of her son's death and during the trial of the perpetrator of this crime. The following illustration demonstrates how to perform a solution-focused safety evaluation.

TABLE 8–4.   Solution-focused questions that evaluate safety issues

- Have you ever been in so much pain that you have considered hurting yourself?
- You must have a good reason for this?
- What has stopped you from acting on these thoughts?
- What else has stopped you?
- What are your reasons for living?
- What else are your reasons for living?
- How confident are you on a scale of 1–10 that you can keep yourself safe?
- What makes it not lower?
- What else makes it not lower?
- What would it take to make it one point higher?
- What else would it take to make it one point higher?
- How confident on a scale of 1–10 are your VIPs that you can keep yourself safe?
- What number would you need to be at to feel confident in your ability to keep yourself safe and not need to go to a higher level of care?
- What number would you need to be at that you would need to go to the emergency room?
- What number would your VIPs say would tell them you need to go to the emergency room?

ANNE: How could I be most helpful for you today?
> *Immediately directing the conversation toward her hopes for the session respectfully places the responsibility for and control of the session in her hands.*

CHRISTINE: I have been feeling suicidal for the past two weeks. I just can't keep going like this.

ANNE: It sounds like things have been really tough for you in the past two weeks. How have you been coping with this?
> *I pair a "for you" response with a coping question.*

CHRISTINE: I don't know. I even wrote a good-bye letter to all my kids.

ANNE: I can see how difficult this has been for you. Did you give the letter to your kids?
> *I explore for a potential positive difference regarding her choice to not give the letter to her children.*

CHRISTINE: No, I didn't give it to them.

ANNE: What stopped you from giving them the good-bye letter?
> *I detail this positive decision.*

CHRISTINE: I couldn't do it to my grandkids. They already lost a father. I just think about wanting to be with my son. It is so painful sometimes that I don't know what to do.

ANNE: I can see how painful this has been for you.
> *The intensity of her pain indicates she needs more "for you" responses.*

CHRISTINE: It has been really horrible. I even had a plan to take all my medications.

ANNE: This must be so painful for you. Did you act on your plan?
>   *I provide an emotional yes-set response and then query whether she acted on this plan.*

CHRISTINE: No.
>   *An important positive difference is discovered.*

ANNE: What stopped you from acting on your plan?
>   *I intentionally begin the safety assessment by asking what stopped her from acting on her plan, choosing to focus on actions that are more constructive.*

CHRISTINE: I thought about my other children and all my grandchildren. They need me.
>   *VIP relationships are discovered and are critical to amplify.*

ANNE: It sounds like you are a very important person in their life. What tells you that your children and grandchildren need you?
>   *I pair a compliment about how important she is to her family with a question. This suggests she is a necessary and indispensable member of her family, further amplifying her VIPs.*

CHRISTINE: My daughter is a new mom and her baby is only one year old. There are a lot of times she really needs my help.

ANNE: What help does your daughter need from you?
>   *I continue to amplify her VIPs and how she is needed in their life.*

CHRISTINE: I watch the baby and help pay for the utilities.

ANNE: She is lucky to have you help her in these ways. I can see how important both she and your grandchild are for you. What else does your daughter need from you?

CHRISTINE: I help her with the rent when she can't afford it.

ANNE: Wow! I am impressed how you are able to help in such important ways, especially given how badly you feel. How are you able to do it?
>   *I provide both direct and indirect compliments.*

CHRISTINE: I love my grandkids, but it's a lot of work. I feel exhausted and can barely get myself out of bed to help.

ANNE: I can see how hard this is for you and how much effort this takes for you. How do you get yourself out of bed when you are feeling so exhausted?
>   *I pair a "for you" response with a coping question.*

CHRISTINE: I just force myself to do it. It makes me get up in the morning and do something.

ANNE: That takes a lot of strength and determination to force yourself to get up in the morning with the way you are feeling. You have such strength to cope with all of this. Where do you get your strength?

CHRISTINE: My grandchildren. I don't want them to have to go through what I went through growing up. I basically raised myself.

ANNE: I can see how important your grandchildren are for you and how much you want them to have a better future. I am wondering, if 10 is you are confident that you can keep yourself safe for your children and grandchildren and 1 is the opposite, where would you say you are now?
>   *I ask scaling questions only after I have discovered and amplified several positive differences, which often increases a patient's hope and confidence.*

CHRISTINE: 5.

ANNE: Is this number going up or down?

CHRISTINE: It's going up.

ANNE: What makes it not lower?

CHRISTINE: I know my daughter needs me, and I want my grandchildren to be a part of my life. I love to see them. I'm hoping to see my grandson in Maine this weekend.

Hopes for future plans are revealed. These are important to amplify.

ANNE: I am impressed with how you are able to make plans to see your other grandson given how difficult things have been for you lately. How are you still able to make plans for yourself, given everything you are coping with?

I provide direct and indirect compliments.

CHRISTINE: I just have to do it. I don't have a choice.

ANNE: That takes tremendous skill and resolve on your part. I am wondering what it would take to make that number go up to a 6, just a little bit better?

CHRISTINE: I will focus on my grandson and going to Maine.

ANNE: That's great. What else will it take to get to a 6?

CHRISTINE: I need to ask my daughter for more help.

This case illustrates how important it is to amplify VIPs and also how useful scaling questions are in evaluating patients for safety. Safety was assessed by asking questions that built on this patient's strengths, VIPs, and resources, and a concrete plan was discussed, all of which could be documented in her chart. As can be seen from this vignette, scaling safety is a particularly useful technique to employ when patients are in crisis.

 Video Illustration: Crisis planning (2:51)

Solution-Focused Assessment of ADHD

Several solution-focused questions help to evaluate ADHD while maintaining a strength-based narrative. Incorporating the phrase "Are you pretty good at..." within the ADHD assessment questions communicates you are confident and assume patients are capable of the behaviors in question. Instead of asking children whether they have trouble concentrating, difficulties listening, or problems with hyperactivity, the solution-focused therapist will instead ask children whether they are "pretty good at" stopping and thinking, paying attention, staying focused, and keeping their body calm. Children are more comfortable answering this positive query and often answer less defensively and more honestly when questions are framed in this way. The question itself conveys that you believe they are pretty good at these skills unless proven otherwise. Another way to ask ADHD questions is by framing the question with "Is it a little bit hard for you to..." and then filling in the blank. For example, is it a little bit hard for you to stop and think, pay attention, or get your homework done? The phrase "a little bit hard" implies that these things may be a "little bit hard," but are not insurmountable and can be overcome. If children say they do have "a little bit of difficulty" with these issues, a solution-focused therapist can follow up with what they have tried to do to manage these challenges and what skills they have used to overcome these difficulties. If they say they don't know or think they don't have the skills, asking them whether they are up for the challenge of learning new skills to overcome these challenges is frequently met with enthusiasm. Children enjoy challenges and want to learn more skills. Learning and mastering skills helps children to gain mastery and self-confidence in their abilities to overcome challenges.

Scaling questions are also helpful in evaluating ADHD. For example, asking patients to rate "how well" they concentrate, focus, get homework done, and stop and think, on a scale of 1–10, can provide a subjective measurement of ADHD. Asking what number their mother, teachers, or other VIPs would rate how well they concentrate, focus, and complete homework takes into account quickly and easily the patient's VIP's perspectives. Table 8–5 lists solution-focused questions to review when assessing ADHD symptoms.

TABLE 8–5. **Solution-focused questions to review in assessment of ADHD symptoms**

- Are you pretty good at concentrating?
- Are you pretty good at listening?
- Are you pretty good at getting your homework done?
- Are you pretty good at stopping and thinking?
- Is it a little bit hard to focus, stop and think, or pay attention?
- How well would you rate your ability to focus on a scale of 1–10?
- How well would you rate your ability to stop and think on a scale of 1–10?
- How well would you rate your ability to keep your body calm on a scale of 1–10?
- What makes it not lower?
- What would make it one point higher?
- How well would your VIPs rate your ability to focus, stop and think, get your homework done, and keep your body calm on a scale of 1–10?

Case Illustration: Solution-Focused Review of Systems in Assessment of ADHD

Tim was a 9-year-old boy whose mother was concerned about whether he had ADHD. He had been diagnosed and treated for ADHD with amphetamine/dextroamphetamine (Adderall), but his mother was concerned whether this was the correct diagnosis and whether his medication was appropriate. She brought in prior evaluations and also revealed that she and her husband had conflicting opinions about the decision to use medications for her son. Tim's evaluation began with an exploration of his strengths, his VIPs, and what he and his mother appreciated about each other. This was followed by eliciting their best hopes for treatment and asking scaling questions. The evaluation then proceeded to the review of systems. Let's look at the review of systems portion of this interview in more detail.

ANNE: I wonder if it would be OK if I ask you some "doctor-type questions" to make sure I have all the information I need to be helpful for you. I know I have already asked a lot of questions, but this will make sure I have not missed anything that may be helpful for you. I ask these questions to all the kids I see. Would this be OK?
I explain the conversational transition and its purpose.

TIM and MOTHER: Yes.

ANNE: Are you pretty good at focusing and paying attention, or is it a little bit hard?
Constructing questions that incorporate positive language helps to sustain a solution-focused conversation.

TIM: It's a little hard.

ANNE: How about getting your homework done? Are you pretty good at this or is it a little bit hard?

TIM: It's a little bit hard.

ANNE: How about staying focused on your work at school, like when there are kids at school talking around you. Are you pretty good at getting your work done in these situations or is it a little bit hard?

TIM: It's hard for me.
Notice how forthcoming and honest he is about his challenges.

ANNE: That must be difficult for you. What about being able to stop and think before you do things? Are you pretty good at that or is it a little bit hard?
Asking whether he is pretty good at stopping and thinking is a positive alternative to asking directly about impulsivity, and is often met with more openness and less defensiveness with children.

TIM: I'm pretty good at that.
An important positive difference is uncovered.

ANNE: That's great. It is hard for a lot of kids to be able to stop and think before they act. Is it helpful for you to stop and think?
A direct compliment is furnished prior to amplifying this positive difference.

TIM: Yes.

ANNE: How is it helpful for you to stop and think?

TIM: I don't want to get into trouble.

ANNE: How else does it help you to stop and think?

TIM: I get to do more things because my mom doesn't take things away.

ANNE: I can see the skill you have at being able to stop and think things through. That's great. What about sleep, do you sleep pretty well at night?
I now move on to further areas of the review of systems.

TIM: Yes.

ANNE: How about eating? Are you a pretty good eater?

TIM: Sometimes the medication makes me not want to eat.

ANNE: This must be difficult for you. How do you manage this?

I bridge a "for you" response with a coping question.

MOTHER: I try to give him a good breakfast, but he doesn't eat anything at lunch and can be pretty irritable when he comes home from school. I try to give him snacks and let him eat at night.

ANNE: You are doing all the right things. It can be difficult for many children to maintain their appetite when taking stimulants. I will make sure to check his weight today. Tim, are you pretty good at calming down?

I provide his mother with more compliments on her parenting ability, while also validating her concerns about her son's weight, and then continue with the review of systems.

TIM: Yes.

ANNE: That's great that you are good at calming down. Calming down is a difficult skill to master. How have you learned how to do this?

I provide a direct and indirect compliment.

TIM: I go and play with Legos or play my video games.

ANNE: How else do you calm down? (*To mother*) Mom, what have done to teach him these skills?

Identifying and amplifying positive differences in children, and then giving parents the credit by asking what they have done to teach their children these skills, simultaneously builds both child and parental competencies.

MOTHER: I work hard to teach him this. I had difficulties learning this as a child, and want to make sure he has these skills.

The vignette illustrates how to obtain necessary information while maintaining a solution-focused conversation. Weaving compliments, emotional validation, coping questions, and preparing patients for questions they will be asked are helpful tools to accomplish this job.

Solution-Focused Assessment of Anxiety

Anxiety is a very common issue for patients. If patients present with this concern, explaining to them that this is not unusual normalizes their experience. Asking patients what they would be doing instead of feeling anxious, scared, or worried guides the conversation toward positive goals. Patients often will say they want to feel more relaxed, get their work done faster, sleep better, or be more able to let things roll off their back. Exploring what patients mean by the word *anxiety* clarifies exactly what this signifies for them in behavioral terms. Asking patients what they have tried to do to manage their anxiety suggests they have been trying to do their best to deal with these difficulties. Solution-focused questions to address anxiety are shown in Table 8–6.

TABLE 8–6.	Solution-focused questions to evaluate anxiety

- How do you manage anxiety?
- How do you cope in these situations?
- On a scale of 1–10, where 10 is you are confident in your abilities to manage your anxiety and 1 is the opposite, where would you say you are?
- How confident would your VIPs say you are, on a scale of 1–10, at managing your anxiety?
- Was it different how you were able to approach that difficult and anxiety provoking situation?
- How was it different?
- Was it helpful?
- How was it helpful?
- How did you have the courage to approach this challenging situation?
- Supposing 10 is you are confident that you could approach this situation again and 1 is the opposite, where would you rate yourself?
- What makes the number not lower?
- What would it take to raise the number by one point?
- What else would it take?

Providing education about anxiety is important in addressing these concerns. Anxiety is a normal feeling and results in characteristic responses for all people. The fight–or–flight response, which causes people to either avoid and run from anxiety or fight back, are quintessential anxiety responses (Clark and Beck 2010). Listening for and inquiring about times patients have approached high-anxiety situations uncovers potential positive differences. Asking whether times when they were able to approach anxiety-ridden situations were different, whether it was helpful for them to approach these situations, and how they had the courage to confront their fears amplifies these positive differences. Asking "how well" patients do at coping with anxiety or managing stressful situations can detect productive strategies they are already having success with. Let's look at a brief example:

> Lizzy was a 7-year-old girl who presented for an evaluation because of parental and school concerns about her level of anxiety. She was struggling each morning to get to school and was visiting the school nurse on a daily basis. In this situation, the solution-focused clinician asked several questions, including her good reasons to go to the nurse and whether it was helpful for her to go to the nurse, and also listened carefully for opportunities to identify and amplify positive differences, such as when her anxiety appeared less and she was able to stay in class without visiting the nurse. Lizzy did have times when she did not visit the school nurse. These times

were amplified by asking her whether this was different, how it was different, whether it was helpful for her, how it was helpful for her, and finally how she did it. She talked about how she would get herself a drink of water from the bubbler, think about recess and how much fun she would have running around with her friends, and focus on her work. She identified these behaviors as helpful for her, and this led to a conversation about what it would take for her to do more of these actions. She was asked to scale her confidence in her ability to continue to do these behaviors from 1–10, and stated she was at a 9. This number was further amplified by asking her what made it not lower, and what else made it not lower. She was then asked what it would take to keep things at a 9. She stated, "Keep doing more of what is working." At the following session, she was maintaining these successful strategies and no longer visiting the school nurse.

Solution-Focused Assessment of Trauma

Traumatic experiences are a sensitive topic for patients and unfortunately are all too common. Prefacing questions that inquire about traumatic experiences by explaining that these questions are asked to everyone during the initial evaluation normalizes this experience for patients. Asking whether patients have ever had to "cope" with traumatic experiences, such as physical abuse, sexual abuse, domestic violence, or other painful losses or experiences suggests the assumption that they would have managed to deal with these distressing circumstances. Incorporating the one word *cope* within the question conveys that the patient has dealt with this suffering, and this communicates their strength, resilience, and courage. This question is very different from asking whether or not a patient has been abused. The solution-focused question implies the working assumption that they have coped in some way with this very painful event in their life.

If patients respond they have coped with abuse or trauma, it is important to first provide enough emotional yes-set responses empathizing with their suffering. It is then critical to bridge this validation with a question asking how they coped with these experiences, and how else they coped. It can also help to scale with them how well they think they have coped with these events on a scale of 1–10. The scale can be amplified in the usual way by asking what makes it not lower and what it would take to raise it by one point.

Yvonne Dolan asks patient who have suffered from trauma to recall times they felt calm, happy, safe, or relaxed, detecting positive differences that can be amplified, thus building their sense of self-efficacy (Y. Dolan, personal communication). Asking patients whether they have had to "cope" with a domestically violent relationship, whether they got out of the relationship, and, if so, how they did this highlights their courage and strength. Solution-focused questions helpful in assessing trauma are listed in Table 8–7.

TABLE 8–7.   Solution-focused questions that are helpful when assessing trauma

- Have you ever had to cope with being physically or sexually abused?
- How did you cope?
- Have you ever had to cope with domestic violence?
- Have you ever had to cope with witnessing domestic violence?
- How did you get out of these relationships?
- How did you cope with these situations?
- How else did you cope?
- Where do you get your strength from to deal with these situations?
- Supposing 10 is you are satisfied with how you are coping and 1 is the opposite, where would you say you are now?
- What makes it not lower?
- What else makes it not lower?
- What would it take to raise it by one point?
- How well would your VIPs say you are coping from 1–10?

Solution-Focused Assessment of Substance Abuse

Substance abuse is a complicated and challenging issue, and for this reason, a whole chapter later in the book (Chapter 10, "Solution-Focused Therapy With Addiction") is devoted to this important issue. The questions outlined here are in no way meant to preclude the many valuable assessment tools used in evaluating substance abuse but are offered with the hope of providing an additive dimension. In asking patients about substance use, it can be helpful to preface questions by affirming that many people have tried using drugs or alcohol, prior to asking if this is something they have experimented with. If they have not tried drugs, what stopped them from doing this? Asking patients what stopped them from using drugs can uncover positive choices and additional useful information, such as not wanting to end up like family members who have suffered from this disease. Asking patients how else they decided to not try drugs can detect additional strengths.

Of course, many times patients will have tried drugs. Especially in working with adolescents, it is important to appreciate their honesty in disclosing this information. People who suffer from addiction often are not forthcoming about their drug use and have good reason to be guarded about their addiction. When patients are honest about their drug use, this is a strength to be acknowledged and appreciated. Beginning by asking how drugs have been helpful for them, and continuing this exploration until no more beneficial aspects of their drug use are revealed, amplifies ambivalence. It is then time to ask how drugs are unhelpful for them, and how else they are unhelpful. Scaling how helpful or unhelpful drugs are for patients, both from their own perspective and their VIPs' perspective, assists in amplifying ambivalence regarding their substance use. Table 8–8 presents solution-focused questions to evaluate substance abuse.

Solution-Focused Assessment of Eating Disorders

Much like the questions asked to assess for ADHD, solution-focused questions to evaluate eating disorders are framed so as to evaluate a patient's body image from a positive direction (Table 8–9).

Solution-Focused Developmental Assessment

Providing patients with a written developmental questionnaire prior to the initial evaluation can help to obtain the necessary information about development without the clinician's needing to spend as much time asking questions to address this domain. Asking patients or parents how old they or their children were when they first became concerned can create a timeline indicating when things were better and what events may have contributed to the presenting concerns. Asking what was different prior to their first concerns, what they tried to do to help manage their concerns, and how they coped with these concerns suggests to patients they are doing all they can to manage.

Solution-Focused Family History Assessment

Obtaining a solution-focused family history can detect resilience, strength, and resources that would otherwise remain undetected. Usually when clinicians think about family history, they are thinking of what diseases and disorders the family has suffered that put the patient at risk for developing these disorders. Asking patients which family members are healthy and doing well, and who in the family does not use drugs or has been successful in recovery, can reveal family resources and additional VIPs that may be of significant help for the patient (Metcalf 2011).

Asking whether family members have "suffered" from depression, substance abuse, anxiety, learning disorders, bipolar illness, or ADHD conveys empathy and can be followed with questions about how these family members have coped with their challenges and what treatments or strategies

TABLE 8–8.	Solution-focused questions to evaluate substance abuse

- Many people have experimented with drugs or alcohol. Is this something you have tried?
- If not: What has stopped you?
- What else has stopped you?

If they have experimented with drugs:

- Are drugs helpful for you?
- How else are they helpful for you?
- How are they unhelpful?
- How else are they unhelpful?
- On a scale of 1–10, where 10 is they are very helpful and 1 is the opposite, how helpful would you rate drugs are for you?
- What makes the number not lower?
- What else makes it not lower?
- On a scale of 1–10, where 10 is they are very unhelpful and 1 is the opposite, how unhelpful would you rate drugs for you?
- How helpful would your VIPs rate your drug use from 1–10, where 10 is they are very helpful for you?
- What is the longest time you have gone without using drugs?
- Was this different for you?
- Was it helpful for you?
- How was it helpful for you?
- How did you do it?
- Were things different between you and your VIPs when you were not using drugs?
- What else was different between you and your VIPs when you were not using?
- How important is it for you on a scale of 1–10 to stay clean and sober?
- How important is it for your VIPs that you stay sober?
- Supposing 10 is you will do anything to keep yourself sober and 1 is the opposite, where would you rate yourself now?
- What makes the number not lower?
- What else makes it not lower?
- What would it take to raise it by one point?
- What else would it take?
- How confident are your VIPs that you can remain sober, where 10 is they are very confident and 1 is the opposite?
- How are things between you and your VIPs on a scale of 1–10 when you are sober?
- How are things between you and your VIPs on a scale of 1–10 when you are using drugs?

TABLE 8–9.   Solution-focused questions to evaluate eating disorders

- Do you feel pretty good about the way you look?
- Supposing 10 is you are satisfied with how your body looks and 1 is the opposite, where would you rate yourself?
- What makes it not lower?
- What else makes it not lower?
- What would it take to raise it one point higher?
- Supposing I asked your VIPs, how healthy would they rate you from 1–10?
- How well are you doing managing your meals from 1–10, where 10 is you are satisfied and 1 is the opposite?
- Supposing I asked your VIPs how well you are managing your meals from 1–10, where 10 is they are satisfied and 1 is the opposite, where do you think they would rate you?
- What makes the number not lower?
- What would they see you doing to raise it by one point?
- Are you "pretty good" at managing your meals or is it "a little bit hard"?
- How are you coping with meals from 1–10, where 10 is you are coping well and 1 is the opposite?

---

have been most helpful for them. Asking what medications have been most helpful for family members can yield very useful information to be considered in choosing medications for patients.

The following excerpt taken from a psychopharmacology assessment of an adolescent, Jacob, who was suffering from anxiety, illustrates how to incorporate solution-focused questions within a family history. The dialog below was between the clinician and Jacob's mother.

Case Illustration: Solution-Focused Family History

ANNE (*addressing Jacob*): First, I need to ask a few "doctor-type" questions to make sure I have not missed any information that would be helpful for me to know prior to prescribing you a medication. Has anyone in your family had to cope with similar difficulties like this?

The word "cope" conveys my belief in the strength of his family. Jacob's mother replies.

MOTHER: I have struggled with anxiety.

ANNE: What has been most helpful for you?

Asking family members what has been most helpful for them quickly directs the conversation toward solutions that have worked for them, providing clues to possible beneficial treatment for other family members.

MOTHER: There was a time I took Prozac [fluoxetine] and that helped, but I don't need it anymore.

ANNE: How was Prozac helpful for you?

Parents who have experienced benefit from a medication are often more willing to try this option for their child.

MOTHER: It helped me function and not feel so depressed. It was especially difficult after Jacob was born. I couldn't even get out of bed. It really helped me be able to function.

ANNE: It sounds like this was a really tough time for you. What else helped you cope with these difficulties?

I continue to pursue all effective treatments of his mother and other family members, hoping this will provide clues as well as a greater willingness, on the part of both Jacob and his parents, to try all possible treatment options that may be beneficial for him.

MOTHER: I saw a therapist for a while, and that really helped, too.

ANNE: Has anyone else in the family coped with anxiety, depression, substance abuse, or other issues you think would be important for me to know?

MOTHER: My mother had some anxiety, but she never got treated for it. It probably would have helped her, but times were different back then.

ANNE: This information is useful because it can help in deciding what medications may be most beneficial for Jacob. Prozac is a very good medication and is a reasonable alternative to try. There are other options such as sertraline or citalopram, but given how helpful Prozac was for you, that seems like a good option for Jacob.

Treatments that are effective for family members are often more easily accepted by children and their parents.

Solution-Focused Rating Scales

Another common tool in the assessment of patients is the use of rating scales. Vast numbers of well-designed standardized testing instruments are available, and these tools allow systematic gathering of information (Dolan 1991; Graham 2007; Leary et al. 2010; Tannock 2008). Most of the current rating scales are used to measure symptom intensity and frequency; however, there is growing interest in strength-based rating scales. Yvonne Dolan (Dolan and 1995) has developed the Solution-Focused Recovery Scale for survivors of sexual abuse. Ron Kral (1995) has developed the Solution Identification Scale for working with children and parents. The Strengths and Difficulties Questionnaire is another scale recognizing a growing interest in the need for these measurements (Vostanis 2006). As examples of how solution-focused scales can be modified for use in assessment, two scales that I have adapted to address issues of ADHD and depression can be reviewed in the Appendix to this book. These scales incorporate positive language and scaling questions as exemplified throughout this book.

LEARNING EXERCISE: SOLUTION-FOCUSED DIAGNOSTIC QUESTIONS

Table 8–10 is a chart divided into diagnostic categories. Complete the chart and then practice asking solution-focused questions that elicit needed diagnostic information in a review of systems, while maintaining a strength-based narrative. Use this chapter to help you with ideas. Share your ideas with colleagues and practice asking these questions to each other to gain fluency with the questions.

KEY POINTS

- The solution-focused clinician does not presume that the solution to a patient's problem is necessarily linked to its cause.

- It is helpful to prepare patients for the change in conversational direction prior to carrying out the review of systems.

- Asking patients how they would rate their mood from 1–10, where 10 is they are satisfied and 1 is the opposite, quickly and easily obtains a subjective assessment of mood.

- Asking patients how things are "between" them and their VIPs from 1–10 can quickly assess the health of important relationships in their life.

- Asking parents to scale how well they remain calm, follow through on limits, and validate their child's experiences with "for you" statements can assess these important parental skills in a nonjudgmental way.

- Asking patients how they calm down, manage frustration, and stop themselves from getting physically aggressive assesses mood while exploring for positive differences.

- Asking patients their "reasons for living" guides the conversation toward hopes, goals, and future dreams.

- When patients have contemplated suicide and not followed through, it is important to ask them what "stopped them" from acting on these thoughts.

- Asking a patient and their VIPs to scale how confident they are that they can keep themselves safe can lead to a collaborative safety plan.

- The solution-focused clinician will assess for ADHD by asking children whether they are "pretty good at" or "is it a little bit hard" for them to stop and think, pay attention, or keep their body calm.

- Listening for times when patients have been able to approach a high-anxiety situation uncovers potential positive differences.

- Asking whether patients have ever had to "cope" with traumatic experiences suggests that, unless the contrary is proven, they have managed to deal with these distressing circumstances.

- When patients are honest about their drug use, this is a strength to be acknowledged and appreciated.

TABLE 8–10.   **Solution-focused diagnostic assessment**

Diagnostic category	Solution-focused review of systems questions
Mood	
Anxiety	
Anger	
ADHD	
Trauma	
Substance abuse	
Eating disorders	
Developmental history	
Psychiatric history	
Family history	

- Asking patients what stopped them from using drugs can uncover positive choices that can be further amplified.

- Asking patients which family members are doing well and which treatments have been most helpful for family members can uncover additional family resources.

References

American Psychiatric Association: American Psychiatric Association Practice Guidelines for the Treatment of Psychiatric Disorders: Compendium 2006. Arlington, VA, American Psychiatric Association, 2006

Clark DA, Beck AT: Cognitive Therapy of Anxiety Disorders: Science and Practice. New York, Guilford, 2010

Coiro MJ, Riley A, Broitman M, et al: Effects on children of treating their mothers' depression: results of a 12-month follow-up. Psychiatr Serv 63:357–363, 2012

Dolan YM: Resolving Sexual Abuse: Solution-Focused Therapy and Ericksonian Hypnosis for Adult Survivors. New York, WW Norton, 1991

Dolan Y, Johnson L: Solution-Focused Recovery Scale for Abuse Survivors. Revised 1995. Available from Y. Dolan (http://www.solutionfocused.net/dolanmain.html)

Dulcan MK: Dulcan's Textbook of Child and Adolescent Psychiatry. Washington, DC, American Psychiatric Publishing, 2010

Fiske H: Hope in Action: Solution-Focused Conversations About Suicide. New York, Routledge/Taylor & Francis Group, 2008

Graham P: Review of assessment scales in child and adolescent psychiatry. Eur Child Adolesc Psychiatry 16:471, 2007

Hales RE, Yudofsky SC: The American Psychiatric Publishing Textbook of Clinical Psychiatry, 4th Edition. Washington, DC, American Psychiatric Publishing, 2003

Hersen M: Psychological Assessment in Clinical Practice: A Pragmatic Guide. New York, Brunner-Routledge, 2004

Kral R: Strategies That Work: Techniques for Solutions in Schools. Milwaukee, WI, BFTC Press, 1995

Leary A, Collett B, Myers K: Rating scales, in Dulcan's Textbook of Child and Adolescent Psychiatry. Edited by Dulcan MK. Washington, DC, American Psychiatric Publishing, 2010, pp 89–110

Metcalf L: Marriage and Family Therapy: A Practice-Oriented Approach. New York, Springer, 2011

Norcross JC, Hogan TP, Koocher GP: Clinician's Guide to Evidence-Based Practices: Mental Health and the Addictions. New York, Oxford University Press, 2008

Simon RI, Hales RE: The American Psychiatric Publishing Textbook of Suicide Assessment and Management. Washington, DC, American Psychiatric Publishing, 2006

Stout CE, Hayes RA: The Evidence-Based Practice Methods, Models, and Tools for Mental Health Professionals. New York, Wiley, 2005

Tannock R: Review of assessment scales in child and adolescent psychiatry. J Child Psychol Psychiatry 49:687, 2008

Vostanis P: Strengths and Difficulties Questionnaire: research and clinical applications. Curr Opin Psychiatry 19:367–372, 2006

Wickramaratne P, Gameroff MJ, Pilowsky DJ, et al: Children of depressed mothers 1 year after remission of maternal depression: findings from the STAR*D-Child study. Am J Psychiatry 168:593–602, 2011

CHAPTER 9

Solution-Focused Psychopharmacotherapy

Psychopharmacotherapy is the combined use of psychoactive medication and psychotherapy, and it requires great skill to execute well. Psychopharmacotherapy has been shown to be effective with many types of patients (Cuijpers et al. 2009a, 2009b; Maalouf and Brent 2012; Otto 2006; Pampallona et al. 2004; Thase 1997). The goal of this chapter is to demonstrate how solution-focused therapy can be utilized in performing psychopharmacotherapy.

Treating patients with psychopharmacological interventions is a complicated, challenging, and rewarding process (Green 2001; Janicak 1997). The psychiatrist is often treating constellations of behavioral symptoms without fully understanding their biological and genetic underpinnings and how they interact with the patient's environment. Developmental issues complicate the use of medications in children because of pharmacokinetic, pharmacodynamic, and neurodevelopmental factors. The long-term effects of medications, and not only psychoactive ones, on growth and development are at best only partially known, and all medications come with side effects. Issues of medication adherence, consent, and assent present additional challenges. Emotions can run high when parents disagree on the use of medications, when the parents are divorced, or when schools are encouraging medications and parents oppose this recommendation. A psychiatrist must be able to successfully negotiate all these difficult issues while maintaining treatment engagement with patients, parents, children, and therapists and attending to protective, legal, and systems issues. To top all this off, psychiatrists often are practicing in a managed care environment in which they are pressured to see patients every 20–30 minutes, usually at best monthly, with the expectation that they will be able to provide magic pharmacological solutions. Needless to say, this is a daunting task!

Paying Attention to the Patient's Hopes and Concerns About Medications

Solution-focused therapy is an extremely helpful skill to bring to the formidable undertaking of effective psychopharmacological treatment. In solution-focused psychopharmacotherapy, it is imperative that patients' wishes and hopes for treatment and their interest in medications remain at the center of the conversation about pharmacotherapy. Listening to, validating, and addressing patients' concerns and questions about medications is an essential first step. Tailoring pharmacotherapy must be done in accordance with patients' best hopes for treatment so that these hopes remain at the center of the conversation, one patient at a time (Sparks et al. 2006). Providing yes-set responses to these concerns, as discussed in previous chapters, helps to maintain and build treatment engagement. Table 9–1 shows some of the questions patients commonly have about medications. These questions must be responded to so that the patient's goals and hopes remain at the center of treatment.

 Video Illustration: Attention to concerns about medications (2:12)

TABLE 9–1.   **Questions patients commonly have about medications**

- Can a medication help with my difficulties?
- Am I taking the right medications?
- What are the long-term consequences of taking a medication?
- What are the risks of medications?
- Is there a medication that can make these problems go away?
- Will I have to take the medication for the rest of my life?
- How long will I have to take medications?
- Is there a blood test for this medication?
- How often will I need to be monitored while taking this medication?
- Will taking medication change my personality?
- Will my child's growth be stunted?
- Will I be dependent on this medication for life?

Just as with other aspects of a solution-focused interview, performing a solution-focused psychopharmacotherapy interview requires asking solution-focused questions. A solution-focused psychopharmacotherapy evaluation begins the same way as any solution-focused interview. It commences with an exploration of problem-free talk, VIPs (very important people), and best hopes for treatment, followed by scaling questions. Table 9–2 presents a list of solution-focused questions adapted for use in a solution-focused psychopharmacotherapy evaluation. These questions preserve the patient at the center of the conversation, maintaining the patient's best hopes, needs, and goals at the forefront of the dialog.

TABLE 9–2. **Questions for use in a solution-focused psychopharma-cotherapy evaluation**

- Suppose there was a magic pill, which we know there isn't, but suppose there was, what are your best hopes as to how the medication would be most helpful for you?
- What would you be doing differently after taking this magic pill?
- What else would you be doing differently?
- What would be different between you and your VIPs when you take this magic pill?
- What would your VIPs notice you doing differently when you take this magic pill?
- What else would your VIPs notice you doing differently?
- Supposing 10 is the medication works like a magic pill and 1 is the opposite, how would you rate the effectiveness of the medication you are taking?
- What number do you think your VIPs would rate the effectiveness of the medication you are taking, from 1–10?
- What makes the number not lower?
- What would make the number higher?
- What percentage do you think it is the medication that is helping, and what percentage is it things you are doing to help the medication work?
- What do you do that helps the medication work?
- What do your VIPs do to help the medication work?
- What medications have you tried that have been most helpful?
- Are there medications that people in your family have tried that have been helpful?

▶ **Video Illustration:** Best hopes for a medication (2:57)

▶ **Video Illustration:** Scaling medication effectiveness (2:25)

▶ **Video Illustration:** Scaling self-efficacy with medications (1:17)

The following case illustrates how to incorporate solution-focused questions when negotiating goals within a psychopharmacological evaluation. In this particular case, both the patient and his parents were very anxious about medication but were also requesting this as a possible treatment option to be explored. They initiated the evaluation with the psychiatrist to discuss their concerns. Utilizing solution-focused approaches can be helpful in these situations. Pay attention to how much time was spent validating the patient's and his parents' concerns, and the solution-focused questions that were asked to maintain their needs and goals at the center of the conversation.

Case Illustration: Solution-Focused Psychopharmacotherapy

Eliot was a 17-year-old boy whose parents brought him for a psychiatric evaluation because of concerns about anxiety. He had suffered from anxiety for many years and had tried therapy, including cognitive-behavioral therapy, with only limited success. His prior treatment providers recommended medication to treat his anxiety, but Eliot and his parents were opposed to pharmacological treatment at that time and had many concerns about medication use. His parents were both well-educated professors and had researched their concerns extensively. Eliot and his parents had tried many things prior to deciding to get a psychiatric consultation, including relaxation exercises, deep breathing, writing anxiety-provoking situations down in a journal, and using herbal remedies. These efforts resulted in some relief, but recent increased stressors caused Eliot's symptoms to worsen. He was having difficulties getting to school and staying in class as a result of experiencing episodes of panic while in the classroom. He would begin to feel physically sick while taking tests, escalating his fears about how he would manage taking college entrance exams. He was reluctant to go on a special trip he had won after receiving high honors in a science competition. He was not sleeping well and was staying up late at night perseverating about the quality of his work, even though he was a straight-A student. His parents were extremely worried about Eliot and didn't know what else to do to help him, so they decided to get a consultation with a psychiatrist to learn more about medication options for their son.

Eliot presented to the initial session as highly anxious and tearful about all his anxieties and how much these symptoms were impairing his function. The initial portion of the interview focused on exploring what Eliot was good at and enjoyed, how he had managed to cope with such severe anxiety, who his VIPs were, and what he appreciated most about them. Eliot had tremendous strengths. He was highly intelligent, hard working, diligent, and goal directed, stayed out of trouble, cared deeply about his family, and was creative and imaginative. His parents cared deeply about their son and were committed to getting him the help he needed. They all came to the appointment prepared with a list of questions and concerns about medications. After spending time exploring, appreciating, and complimenting their strengths and VIPs, I began goal negotiation. The following vignette begins at this juncture in the interview.

ANNE: How could I be most helpful for you so that this meeting today is worthwhile for you?

ELIOT: I want to know if there is a medication that can help me with all the anxiety I have been feeling. I just can't stand feeling this way anymore.

Notice that it was the patient who initiated the conversation regarding medications.

ANNE: This must be so difficult for you. I can see all the ways you have been working so hard to try and cope with your anxiety. You don't give up. Supposing there was a magic pill that could take away your anxiety, which we know there isn't, but suppose there was, what would you be doing differently?

I bridge a "for you" response and compliment with the "magic pill" question to define his best hopes about medications.

ELIOT: I wouldn't be having all this anxiety. I wouldn't be scared to go to school because I'm worried about getting sick in class.

ANNE: What would you be doing instead when you no longer are experiencing this anxiety?

ELIOT: I don't know (*pause*). I'd be able to get up more easily in the morning and go to school without feeling sick.

My first response is to pause and give him more time to think about this question, keeping the conversational ball in his court. My patience paid off.

ANNE: What else would you be doing?

ELIOT: I'd be able to stay in class without worrying about having a panic attack.

ANNE: What else would you be doing?

ELIOT: I'd be able to take a test without having to leave the classroom.

ANNE: What else would you be doing?

ELIOT: I'd be able to go on class trips without freaking out about my anxiety.

ANNE: What else would you be doing?

ELIOT: I don't know. That would be a lot.

He can no longer reveal further details, indicating it is timely to move on to different questions.

ANNE (*asking parents*): What would you notice Eliot doing differently after taking this magic pill?

I now ask his parents, expanding the goals to incorporate his VIPs' perspectives.

FATHER: He would get to sleep at a reasonable time without staying up so late doing homework.

ANNE: What else would he be doing?

FATHER: We would not fight about him going to bed at night. I get so worried about his lack of sleep that I force him to go to bed. He gets angry thinking that I don't want him to succeed. This isn't true at all. I know he will do well. I just want him to be able to have some fun and enjoy his life too. I don't want him to stay home because of all his anxiety, when he could go on this great trip and have fun with his friends.

ANNE: This sounds like it has been very difficult for all of you. I am impressed with how hard you have all been working to help Eliot cope and manage his anxiety. Eliot asked about medication options. There are medications available that could help his anxiety. These are used in combination with therapy and can help Eliot develop the skills he has already been using to cope with his anxiety. Would this be of interest to you?

Providing suggestions in the form of a question maintains a collaborative conversation.

FATHER: I am concerned about all the side effects and whether it would be the right thing for Eliot.

It is important to address and validate parental medication concerns. Parents are vital in encouraging, monitoring, dispensing, and paying for medication. Building a strong alliance with parents is critical for effective treatment with children.

ANNE: I can tell how much you have thought about this, and how concerning this is for you. These are difficult decisions to make. What would tell you that a medication is the right thing for Eliot?

This question conveys my respect and interest in learning about his father's ideas about medications, further strengthening parental treatment engagement.

FATHER: That he wouldn't be suffering so much of the time. Things have gotten pretty bad at home. He's not sleeping, he's crying, he's worrying, and he seems to be spinning his wheels.

ANNE: I can see how deeply you care about Eliot, and how worried you are for him. This must be very concerning for you. What do you think he would be doing differently supposing he got the right medication?

I provide more compliments and "for you" statements prior to asking another question to explore his father's hopes for medications.

FATHER: He would get his work done when he gets home from school rather than worrying about doing it and feeling anxious. It is not unusual that it's nine o'clock at night when he begins his work. He would be able to get to sleep at a reasonable hour and not be so exhausted in the morning making things even worse.

His father formulates more positively worded, realistic, and measurable goals.

ANNE: What else would he be doing differently?

I continue this exploration asking what else.

MOTHER: He wouldn't call from school in a panic that he was sick, and he would be able to get through his day more easily. I hope he would have more fun.

ANNE: What would he be doing when is more able to have fun?

I continue to ask questions that specify his goals.

MOTHER: He would be able to go on the trip he won and not be so anxious about getting sick on the bus. He gets so worried about getting sick that he doesn't go out and do fun things.

ANNE: That must be disappointing for him. What else would he be doing?
ELIOT: I wouldn't wake up in the morning feeling so worried about getting
  sick in school.
  Eliot adds to the goals but formulates them negatively.
ANNE: What would you be doing instead?

This case illustrates how asking solution-focused questions maintains patients and their VIPs at the center of the conversation, specifying goals that they have determined would indicate that treatment is effective for them, while building treatment engagement and acquiring the necessary information for effective treatment. Intense feelings often emerge when medications are discussed. These were critical to validate by providing emotional yes-set responses, as was guiding the conversation toward solutions by asking useful questions. Attending to both Eliot's and his VIPs' concerns and dialog was a critical step in this process. Of utmost importance is that the focus of treatment remains on the patient and his or her best hopes for the preferred future. Eliot was seen several weeks later, having tried the medication that was prescribed. Eliot and both his parents were very pleased with how helpful the medication was for him. This conversation was instrumental in facilitating treatment adherence for Eliot and his VIPs.

Solution-focused therapy can also be helpful in high-conflict situations. Sustaining a positive, solution-focused conversation can be especially difficult when there is hostility. The following case illustrates how to use solution-focused therapy with divorced parents who are experiencing a high amount of discord concerning the issue of medication for their son. Pay attention to how the therapist guided the session during these moments by preceding solution-focused questions with compliments and emotional yes-set responses, mindfully incorporating the participants' language with the statements and questions. The therapist remained vigilant to the patient's emotional needs by providing emotional yes-set responses and paid heed to all possible opportunities to bestow compliments. These responses were promptly followed with solution-focused questions that preempted potential acrimony and antipathy, instead steering the dialog toward the patient's and family's needs and best hopes for treatment.

Case Illustration: Solution-Focused Psychopharmacotherapy in a High-Conflict Situation

Jeff was a 7-year-old boy who was being treated for attention-deficit/hyperactivity disorder (ADHD). His parents, Helen and Bill, were divorced, and although his father was invited to his sessions, he chose not to come, stating issues with how far the appointments were from his home and conflicts with his work schedule. Jeff received the diagnosis of ADHD through a comprehensive psychological and psychiatric evaluation, including a school assessment. He was treated with extended-release methylphenidate (Ritalin LA) and was doing moderately well except for some loss of appetite. Things were going well until his mother called concerned that when Jeff was visiting his father over the weekend, his father told Jeff that he didn't need medications. Jeff became anxious and spoke to his mother. His mother became very angry with his father and called to express her concern about how to handle this situation. She was concerned that his father was sabotaging Jeff's treatment, which she had worked so hard to get for her son. Jeff's father was invited to the next appointment. The following is an excerpt from this session.

ANNE: Thank you both for coming. I realize this is a long trip for you (*addressing Bill*). I really appreciate you taking the time to come and arranging your work schedule to make this happen.
Thanking people conveys they are part of the solution.
BILL: I would do anything for Jeff.
ANNE: Of course. I am wondering what you most appreciate about Jeff?
I commence the conversation by directing questions toward what his father appreciates about Jeff, making parental conversational deposits.
BILL: I just love when he comes to visit. He lights up my weekend.
ANNE: Wow! That's wonderful. What does he do to light up your weekend?
BILL: I don't really know. I think it's just who he is.
ANNE: I can see how much you enjoy your son. What do you enjoy doing with Jeff?
I continue pursue more details about the positive aspects of their relationship.
BILL: We play Legos together, and we also play basketball.
ANNE: What else do you enjoy doing with him?
BILL: We try to do fun things together when he visits, like biking. He also really loves spending time with his grandmother and aunt.
ANNE: What else do you appreciate about him?
BILL: He loves to help, and he is always willing to help his grandmother.
ANNE: That's wonderful. Where does he get this quality?
BILL: I don't know, probably from his mother, and maybe a little from me.
He compliments his ex-wife and also himself, directing the conversation in a positive direction.
ANNE: What does he get from you?
BILL: I work in the military and teach classes. I like to help people learn new things.
ANNE: That sounds like challenging work. What kind of work do you do in the military?
People's jobs and professions are important areas to explore for strengths and resources.
BILL: I had two tours in Iraq. It was challenging. I was away a lot when Jeff was young, and I think that may have affected him.
ANNE: That is impressive. That must take tremendous dedication, courage, and commitment.
BILL: Yes.
ANNE: I'm wondering how I could be most helpful for you both, so that this meeting is useful for the two of you and you can say it was worthwhile to come?

I embark on goal negotiation questions only after enough conversational deposits have been made.

BILL: I worry that Jeff doesn't interact with others. He takes a while to start talking and has a hard time listening. He always seems to want to negotiate everything.

ANNE: I can tell you have thought a lot about this. What are your best hopes for this meeting today so it will be worthwhile for you?

BILL: I just want him to get the help he needs and be sure this medication is really helping him.

ANNE: Of course, it sounds like you've thought about this a lot. And what about you (*turning to Helen*), what are your best hopes for this meeting today?

It is important that each parent have time to voice their hopes for the meeting so goals can be negotiated in a collaborative way.

HELEN: I just want us to be on the same page with the medications. I was so worried this weekend when I heard from Jeff that you told him he should try to do all this on his own. It seemed like he had to almost beg for you to give him his medications.

ANNE: Of course, this must have been worrying and frustrating for you. What do you mean "on the same page"?

HELEN: That we are communicating and that we are telling Jeff the same thing. I want his dad to know that it was very difficult to get to this point. I worked so hard to get him treatment and waited years before trying medication, and then for him to just do this—tell Jeff he didn't need medication. I was furious.

ANNE: Of course, this must have been very frustrating for you.

Given the power of Helen's affect, it is important to provide an emotional yes-set response. Prematurely asking questions at this point may cause her to feel dismissed.

HELEN: Yes (*appearing tearful*).

ANNE: What do you need from Bill that would tell you that you are on the same page?

When patients are very upset, it may indicate there is an unmet need. Asking what she needs from Bill maintains the conversation in a positive direction.

HELEN: I need him to communicate with me before doing things like this. I need him to talk with me and if he has concerns to check things out, so Jeff is not put in the middle of all this.

ANNE: Of course, this makes sense. And (*addressing Bill*) what do you need from Helen?

I validate Helen's concerns and then ask Bill what he needs from Helen. In this way I am attending to both of their needs, preventing the conversation from deteriorating into a blame game.

BILL: I just want to be told what's going on. I want to make sure this medication is right for Jeff.

ANNE: Of course, it is important to know that the medication your child is receiving is helpful for them. Is there any information you need from me that would help you know this is the right medication for him?

I explore any medication concerns he has.

BILL: Does he really need this medication?

ANNE: Based on his extensive testing, history, and response to the medication he is on, he appears to be getting a lot of benefit from this medication. Medications for ADHD have been studied for many years and have a lot of evidence to back their effectiveness. He does have some appetite loss, which I am monitoring closely. The reports from school also indicate he has responded very well to this medication. Of great importance is that Jeff himself indicates the medication is very helpful for him. Are there any other concerns that you have?

BILL: I just need to know what's going on and have his mother include me more.

HELEN: I do tell you. I have invited you to every IEP [Individualized Education Program] meeting and every therapy session. I don't call you every day with every little thing, but I can't do that. I work full-time and it would drive me crazy.

ANNE: Of course, this must be frustrating for you, and I can see how hard you are working to keep Bill informed. I'm wondering if I could ask you both a number question. This number question would help me better help you. Suppose I have a scale between 1–10 where 10 is you are satisfied that you are on the same page and 1 is the opposite. Where would you say you are now?

At this point, it would be very easy for the conversation to quickly deteriorate. I need to take control while also making sure I validate their concerns. I begin by providing Helen an emotional yes-set response and compliment followed with a scaling question. Scaling questions are extremely helpful in keeping the conversation calm and goal directed.

HELEN: 3 to 4.

ANNE (*looking at Bill*): And how about for you, what number would you say things are at in terms of being on the same page?

BILL: 3 to 4.

ANNE: What makes this number not lower than a 3 to 4?

BILL: I know she does call and does try to communicate with me. I just want her to call me more about how he does in school.

HELEN: I do communicate with you about his school meetings and major issues he has, like if he is called to the principal's office. I don't call you with every concern. I don't have time. I work full-time. You can always call the school yourself. And when I do ask you to come to school meetings, you usually don't come. I worry about what you say to him. I know you have told me you're concerned that he will turn into a drug addict with these pills and that you do have an issue with these medications, but you don't talk to me about it. I just want you to talk to me about these concerns; otherwise you put him in the middle. It's about what Jeff needs.

ANNE: Of course, these are important concerns and important to address. I am wondering what makes the number not lower for you regarding your communication?

I maintain the focus on scaling questions.

HELEN: I know he really cares about Jeff and know he wants to be involved. I just get so frustrated when he does things like tell him not to take his medication. I have worked so hard to get Jeff the help he needs and I would think Bill would appreciate it. I do this because I don't want Jeff to struggle like you have. Both you and your brother have ADHD and nothing was ever done. I don't want to have him struggle like you did.

Notice how the scaling question keeps the conversation productive.

ANNE: You work very hard, have thought a lot about Jeff's needs, and care deeply. What would it take to make it a 4?

HELEN: That Bill would talk to me first about any questions with the medications, so it doesn't go through Jeff, putting him in the middle.

ANNE: Of course, that makes a lot of sense. What else would make it a 4?

HELEN: That he would come to some of the therapy sessions, school conferences, and school events, and not just tell him the medications are bad without talking with me.

ANNE (*addressing Bill*): What would it take to get to a 4 for you?

BILL: I think calling and coming to more appointments, like she said, would help… I do think they are helpful. It helps to get my questions answered and have a place that we can talk together. I could do it as long as I get advance notice.

ANNE: That's great. I am so impressed with how hard the two of you are working on Jeff's behalf. It takes a lot of dedication, commitment, and love, which you both clearly have. Supposing 10 is you are very confident you can take these next steps to get yourself on the same page, and one is the opposite, how confident are you that you will be able to take these next steps to get more on the same page with your communication?

HELEN: I would say a 6.

BILL: I would say an 8.

ANNE: That's fantastic. What gives you this confidence?

BILL: I think the fact we are here together talking and coming up with ideas has been very helpful. We already do a lot together, and that gives me confidence.

ANNE: And what about you, what gives you confidence you have what it takes to move things forward in your communication so you are on the same page?

HELEN: I am glad Bill came today. It really helps when we have time to talk and figure out a plan. I think my confidence will grow more when I see that he calls Jeff more regularly and comes to more appointments with me.

This conversation illustrates how solution-focused therapy can be helpful in working with people who are in conflict, and is especially important in working with parents who have differing opinions about medications for their children. The conversation attended to both parents' needs and best hopes for treatment, keeping them and their son's needs as the focal point of treatment.

LEARNING EXERCISE: PSYCHOPHARMACOTHERAPY

Imagine a patient who is being treated with medications. On a scale of 1-10, where 10 is you (the clinician) are very satisfied that you have done everything possible to achieve rapport in order to encourage, support, and motivate the patient to behave in ways that will optimize the patient's adherence to medication, and 1 is the opposite, where would you rate yourself? Where do you suppose the patient would rate your helpfulness in regard to his or her medication treatment? What is the reason the number is not lower? What else makes it not lower? What would it take to raise it by one point? What else would it take to raise it by one point?

KEY POINTS

- Just as in other solution-focused conversations, in performing pharmacotherapy it is important to commence with problem-free talk, an exploration of a patient's VIPs, and best hopes for the session.

- Listening to and appreciating a patient's concerns and questions about medications is an important first step in performing pharmacotherapy.

- Asking patients their "best hopes" for a medication is a useful question in negotiating goals for pharmacotherapy treatment.

- Scaling questions can quickly evaluate medication effectiveness from multiple perspectives while also facilitating next steps and goal negotiation.

- Asking patients what percentage of their progress is due to the medications and what percentage is due to them can enhance their self-efficacy while simultaneously building treatment adherence.

- Scaling questions are helpful to use in high-conflict situations and can assist the clinician in guiding the conversation in a productive fashion.

References

Cuijpers P, Dekker J, Hollon SD, et al: Adding psychotherapy to pharmacotherapy in the treatment of depressive disorders in adults: a meta-analysis. J Clin Psychiatry 70:1219–1229, 2009a

Cuijpers P, van Straten A, Warmerdam L, et al: Psychotherapy versus the combination of psychotherapy and pharmacotherapy in the treatment of depression: a meta-analysis. Depress Anxiety 26:279–288, 2009b

Green WH: Child and Adolescent Clinical Psychopharmacology. Philadelphia, PA, Lippincott Williams & Wilkins, 2001

Janicak PG: Principles and Practice of Psychopharmacotherapy. Baltimore, MD, Williams & Wilkins, 1997

Maalouf FT, Brent DA: Child and adolescent depression intervention overview: what works, for whom and how well? Child Adolesc Psychiatr Clin N Am 21:299–312, 2012

Otto MW: Combined psychotherapy and pharmacotherapy for mood and anxiety disorders in adults: review and analysis. FOCUS 4:204–214, 2006

Pampallona S, Bollini P, Tibaldi G, et al: Combined pharmacotherapy and psychological treatment for depression: a systematic review. Arch Gen Psychiatry 61:714–719, 2004

Sparks JA, Duncan BL, Miller SD: Integrating psychotherapy and pharmacotherapy: myths and the missing link. Journal of Family Psychotherapy 17: 83–108, 2006

Thase ME: Integrating psychotherapy and pharmacotherapy for treatment of major depressive disorder. Current status and future considerations. J Psychother Pract Res 6:300–306, 1997

CHAPTER 10

Solution-Focused Therapy
With Addiction

Treating people who suffer from addiction is a challenging and rewarding endeavor. Solution-focused therapy is a very beneficial skill to incorporate into addiction treatment and has been written about extensively (Anderson and Goolishian 1991; Berg 1996; Berg and Miller 1992; Berg and Shafer 2004; de Shazer and Isebaert 2004; McCollum and Trepper 2001; Pichot 2001; Pichot and Smock 2009; Yeager and Gregoire 2005). Many people who have this disease, especially those who are adolescents, are externally motivated (mandated) into treatment. Often people with addiction suffer from myriad other problems, including co-occurring disorders that make dual diagnosis the norm rather than the exception (Minkoff 2001). Patients with addiction are often ambivalent about stopping their substance use, and their very important people (VIPs) are exhausted from having been subjected to the pernicious effects of this malignant disease. Both patients and their VIPs are in extreme need of comfort, support, and help.

Using solution-focused therapy with those suffering from addiction involves using the same skills discussed throughout this book: beginning the conversation by identifying and magnifying strengths through the amplification of positive differences, discovering VIPs and what is most appreciated about them, negotiating best hopes for treatment, asking the miracle question, and harnessing scaling questions. Maintaining a yes-set, providing plenty of compliments, incorporating a patient's language within the questions, and taking a curious and nonassuming stance are employed, just as with other patients.

Commencing With Strengths

Commencing with strengths is especially important in treatment of patients who suffer from addiction. Discovering positive differences and capturing as many opportunities as possible to compliment patients early on and throughout the conversation builds engagement while increasing self-efficacy (Berg and De Jong 2005; Campbell et al. 1999). It is these very strengths that will be conducive to recovery. Even when patients are unable to identify strengths in areas outside their drug use, they often have many well-developed skills that they exploit when obtaining drugs and sustaining their drug habit. Beginning by complimenting their skills, even if these are related to their drug use, accumulates indispensable conversational deposits. For example, one patient responded to being asked what she is good at by talking about all the ways she is able to buy and sell drugs. Complimenting her entrepreneurial spirit, ability to make connections, and courage laid the groundwork that these were all skills that could be redirected toward positive means. Especially in working with externally motivated patients, finding ways to provide genuine compliments is critical to building engagement. Paying attention to positive differences is paramount. Such differences may include times when patients are able to have periods of abstinence (even if very brief), manage drug cravings, acknowledge and experience intense feelings without relapsing, get back on track after a relapse, stop and think through the consequences of their actions, attend a 12-step meeting, call and reach out to their supports or sponsors, do the next right thing, accomplish parts of their goals, and consider how their actions would affect their loved ones.

The following case exemplifies the importance of beginning with strengths. This practice is particularly important with people with multiple problems that could easily lead both the patient and the clinician to feel defeated. Notice that commencing with strengths exposes tremendous resilience, talents, and assets in what could otherwise feel like a hopeless case. When reading the following vignette, notice the order of questions: beginning with strengths and VIPs in problem-free talk, then continuing to goal negotiation and scaling questions. Notice that the patient's words were integrated within the questions and plenty of "for you" responses and compliments were provided. Notice that positive differences were listened for and amplified, and that scaling questions were then asked to further magnify strengths and clarify goals.

Case Illustration: Starting With Strengths in Addiction

Michael was a 22-year-old man who was being treated at a rehabilitation center for drug addiction. He required a psychiatric evaluation to assess his diagnosis and to provide treatment recommendations. He had been living with his adoptive father. Prior to his admission, he was treated at a detoxification facility. He had two prior psychiatric hospitalizations in the past year for suicide attempts. He was on probation for drug possession charges. Michael had a long and traumatic past history, beginning with in utero heroin exposure. He was removed from the care of his biological mother to a foster home when he was very young and then later adopted. His adoptive mother suffered from severe alcohol dependence and was dying from cirrhosis of the liver. He moved in with his adoptive father at age 12 because his adoptive mother was unable to care for his needs. His adoptive father also suffered from alcohol dependence and had become sober only recently, at the time of Michael's current admission. Michael reported a long history of physical and sexual abuse. Although he had many half-siblings, none were described as helpful or supportive. Michael was diagnosed with myriad psychiatric conditions, including attention-deficit/hyperactivity disorder (ADHD), bipolar disorder, posttraumatic stress disorder (PTSD), generalized anxiety disorder, attachment disorder, and a significant learning disability, and was currently prescribed multiple medications.

ANNE: I appreciate your talking with me today. I hope I can be helpful for you. In order to do that, I will need to ask you some questions. Some of these questions can be very hard. Would this be OK?

MICHAEL: Yes.

ANNE: I will try my best, and hope you will, too.

MICHAEL: OK.

ANNE: What are some things that you enjoy or are good at?

MICHAEL: I like to draw.

ANNE: Great. What do you like to draw?

MICHAEL: Animals.

ANNE: What kinds of animals do you like to draw?

MICHAEL: Birds.

ANNE: Wow! They sound like they are difficult to draw. How did you become interested in drawing birds?

MICHAEL: I have birds at home.

ANNE: Really? Wow! What kinds of birds do you have at home?

MICHAEL: I have a parrot, two mourning doves, and a parakeet.

ANNE: Wow! That's a lot of birds. That must take a lot of expertise to handle all these kinds of birds.

MICHAEL: I don't know. I've just always had birds.

ANNE: What does it take to care for birds?

MICHAEL: They are not that hard to take care of. My parrot can talk and say some words.

ANNE: Wow! How did you manage to teach it to talk?

MICHAEL: You just practice with them. My mourning doves like to play with me.

ANNE: Really. Mourning doves play with you? They must be so smart. How do you play with birds?

MICHAEL: I let them out of the cage and put little bells and places for them to hide. They like when I chase them around the house.

ANNE: That's fantastic! Where did you learn how to take care of birds?

MICHAEL: My mom. I mean my adoptive mom. She always had birds. We've always had a lot of animals at home.

ANNE: That's great. Do you have other animals at home as well?

MICHAEL: Two dogs, two cats, and two snakes.

ANNE: Wow! Two snakes! What kind of snakes do you have?

MICHAEL: An albino corn snake and a ball python.

ANNE: That must take a lot to take care of all of them.

MICHAEL: Not really. It's pretty easy. The ball python likes to curl up on my lap and then it just unravels itself when it feels comfortable. They like to annoy my cats.

ANNE: Really? How do the snakes annoy your cats?

MICHAEL: They come out and hiss at them. It's pretty funny.

ANNE: Wow! Your house sounds amazing.

The conversation began with problem-free talk. It centered on uncovering as many details as possible in these areas, conveying his expertise in drawing and in caring for and training animals, practicing, and learning skills. Many conversational deposits were made, and these are especially critical when available resources appear minimal.

Identifying a patient's VIPs and what they most appreciate about them is especially critical in treating those with addiction. The harmful effects of addiction have often devastated many of their relationships. It is imperative to discover all of a patient's VIPs, because these relationships will be paramount for their recovery. Inviting them to talk about what they most appreciate about their VIPs accrues vital relationship deposits for the patient, while strengthening bonds that have often been severely damaged from the disease of addiction.

Let's continue with the prior case, illustrating an exploration of Michael's VIPs.

ANNE: I'm wondering who are the most important people in your life?

MICHAEL: My father (*referring to his adoptive father*). There are a lot of people in my life, but he's the only one who has really been there for me.

ANNE: What do you most appreciate about your father?

MICHAEL: He is always there. He has never let me down.

ANNE: What has he done to never let you down?

MICHAEL: He always tries to help me and tells the truth, even if I don't like to hear it.

ANNE: What else do you appreciate about him?

MICHAEL: He has taught me a lot.

ANNE: What has he taught you?

MICHAEL: He works in landscaping. I've been mowing lawns since I was three years old.

ANNE: Wow! That's amazing! What else has he taught you?

MICHAEL: I know a lot about flowers.

ANNE: Tell me about the flowers you know about.

MICHAEL: My favorite is morning glories. We planted tons of them.

ANNE: Wow! What else do you know about planting?

MICHAEL: I know all about fruit trees. My father has a mini-orchard and he has taught me how to prune apple trees, pear trees, grapes, and peach trees.

ANNE: That's fantastic. You have a lot of skills.

MICHAEL: I used to sell fruits in front of my house. And sometimes even the crafts I made.

ANNE: What kinds of crafts did you make?

MICHAEL: I would make all sorts of things. My grandmother taught me how.

ANNE: Your grandmother sounds like an important person in your life.

MICHAEL: She was, but she died two years ago.

ANNE: I'm sorry. That must be difficult for you. How have you coped with this?

MICHAEL: I cope by taking long walks in the forest near where I live.

ANNE: Is that helpful for you?

MICHAEL: Yes.

ANNE: How does it help you?

MICHAEL: I get to hear the sounds of birds and feel safe among the trees. It reminds me of when I would spend the days on the beach with my mother playing. It makes me forget about things.

ANNE: How else do you cope?

MICHAEL: I cook with my father.

ANNE: Wow! What do you like to cook with your father?

MICHAEL: Anything—eggs, vegetables, anything from our garden. He likes to use herbs.

ANNE: Sounds wonderful. How else do you cope?

MICHAEL: I like to skip rocks in the pond nearby. I'm pretty good.

ANNE: I bet. Where did you learn how to skip rocks?

MICHAEL: From my father, he's taught me everything.

ANNE: I am amazed by all the skills and things you have learned from your father and how you have coped with all the challenges you have faced. You have been here about one month, and I'm wondering what has been better since you have been here?

Notice that with an exploration of his VIPs, further relational strengths were identified, as were his coping abilities. Michael obviously has tremendous resilience to have handled all the difficult life experiences he has been dealt. Focusing on these strengths and coping abilities early is crucial. I conclude the conversation by asking "what's better" as a transition point to guide the dialogue toward goal negotiation.

Goal Negotiation and Amplifying Ambivalence in Addiction

The next step is goal negotiation, which often begins by amplifying patients' ambivalence about their drug use. Rather than directly confronting a patient's denial, asking patients their "good reasons" for using drugs, and how drugs are helpful for them, respectfully explores their motivation to use drugs. These questions convey that they are the expert on their good reasons for using drugs, while generating and sustaining an agreeable conversational direction. After pursuing all the details of how drugs are helpful and all their good reasons for using drugs, patients eventually admit that drugs are unhelpful. If they don't acknowledge this, asking patients whether their VIPs view drugs as helpful or unhelpful assists in amplifying their ambivalence. Scaling how helpful and unhelpful drugs are, from both the patient's and their VIPs' perspectives, can further magnify ambivalence (Table 10–1).

TABLE 10–1.   Questions that amplify ambivalence in addiction

- You must have a good reason to use drugs?
- How helpful are drugs for you?
- How else are they helpful for you?
- How helpful are drugs for you on a scale of 1–10, where 10 is most helpful and 1 is the opposite?
- How helpful would your VIPs say drugs are for you from 1–10?
- How unhelpful would your VIPs say drugs are for you from 1–10?
- How much do you want to stay sober from 1–10?
- How much do you need to stay sober from 1–10?
- What makes the number not lower?
- What else makes it not lower?
- How much would your VIPs say you need to stay sober from 1–10?
- How confident are you that you can remain sober from 1–10?
- How confident are your VIPs that you can remain sober from 1–10?
- What makes it not lower?
- What else makes it not lower?
- What would it take to raise it by one point?

Amplifying ambivalence can also be fostered by asking patients whether they are currently accomplishing their plans. The plans of people with addiction are frequently coming to naught. Instead of trying to convince patients about the unhelpfulness of their drug problem, inquiring with them whether it was in their plans to be in rehab, to be failing school, to be on probation, or to have lost their friends and family often elicits negative replies. These questions stimulate patients to contemplate how their choices are affecting what they want or don't want in their life, and what they want to do differently, while maintaining the yes-set. Asking patients what their VIPs would notice them doing differently when they are succeeding with their plans spells out in greater detail their goals. A good sign that people are working on their recovery is that their plans are coming to fruition.

Asking patients about their best hopes for treatment and how the clinician can be most helpful so that meeting with the clinician is worthwhile for them is a way to proceed with goal negotiation. This query can be met with a variety of responses—anything from desperately wanting help to getting their probation officer or parents off their back, being able to go back home with their family, keeping their marriage together, regaining their driver's license, getting a job, winning trust back, or improving relationships with their VIPs. Asking patients what would it take for this to happen, and what else it would take, are additional questions that expound their goals. Scaling how satisfied they are that they are meeting their goals on a scale of 1–10 acquires their perspective on whether they are achieving their hopes and aspirations. Asking what makes it not lower and what it would take to raise this number elaborates specific steps they can take to fulfill their goals. The following case illustrates solution-focused techniques to negotiate goals in an externally motivated patient.

Case Illustration: Goal Negotiation With an Externally Motivated Patient

Jenny was a 15-year-old girl who was mandated into treatment by her probation officer following assault and battery charges. She was transferred from youth detention after being there for the past 6 months. She had been in and out of foster care for the past 2 years and had suffered trauma after witnessing severe chronic domestic violence between her parents that resulted in her father being incarcerated. She had seen numerous treatment providers and had been tried on multiple medications. She presented to the rehabilitation center suffering from multiple drug addictions, including daily cannabis, nicotine, alcohol, PCP, Percocet, and ecstasy use. The following is an excerpt from an initial interview after she had been in treatment for a few days. Notice that positive differences were explored and amplified prior to goal negotiation. Asking questions in this order offers more opportunities to compliment patients, which is particularly important in externally motivated patients.

ANNE: Hi, Jenny. I appreciate your meeting with me today. I was asked to talk with you to see how I could be helpful. In order to help you, I ask a lot of questions, and some of them can be very difficult. Would it be OK if I asked you a few questions to see how we may be most able to help you?

JENNY: Sure.

ANNE: What has been better since you have been here?

JENNY: I haven't exploded yet.

ANNE: What do you mean exploded?

JENNY: I haven't punched anyone yet.

ANNE: Is that different for you?

JENNY: Yes.

ANNE: How is that different?

JENNY: I've been in lock-up six times for that. I used to do whatever.

ANNE: What are you doing instead of exploding?

JENNY: I'm thinking before I react.

ANNE: Is that different?

JENNY: Yes.

ANNE: Has it been helpful for you?

JENNY: Yes.

ANNE: How has it been helpful for you?

JENNY: I'm staying out of trouble.

ANNE: How have you been able to do this?

JENNY: If I explode, there's no other option but being put back into lock-up.

ANNE: And this option to go back to lock-up, is this the option you want?

JENNY: No. Lock-up is not an option.

ANNE: Is this different for you that lock-up is no longer an option?

JENNY: Yeah. I know what it's like now. I couldn't even wear my own clothes there. I don't want to see that place ever again.

ANNE: What do you want to see instead?

JENNY: My house and my mother.

ANNE: So you want to get back to your house with your mother?

JENNY: Yes.

ANNE: What will it take for you to get back to your house?

JENNY: I have to do what's right. Stay in school and stay sober.

ANNE: Is this different that you want to do what's right and stay sober?

JENNY: Yes. I used to not care.

ANNE: Is it different that you care now?

JENNY: Yeah.

ANNE: How is it different?

JENNY: I can see the brighter side of myself.

ANNE: How did you learn to see the brighter side of yourself?

JENNY: I haven't run from here and I am following directions. I'm learning I am capable.

ANNE: What else tells you that you are capable?

JENNY: I'm actually trying to listen.

ANNE: Is that different that you are listening?

JENNY: Yes. I'm actually trying to think about what people tell me.

ANNE: Is that different?

JENNY: Yes.

ANNE: How is it different?

JENNY: I want to change. I don't want to go back to my old ways.

ANNE: What do you mean old ways?

JENNY: Using and all that old behavior that got me into lock-up. Not caring. Angry.

ANNE: Supposing 10 is you are confident that you will not go back to your old ways and 1 is the opposite, where would you say you are now?

JENNY: 8.

ANNE: What is the reason it is not lower?

JENNY: I'm not as angry.

ANNE: How have you been managing your anger differently?

JENNY: I take space.

ANNE: What else?

JENNY: I keep busy.

ANNE: What do you do to keep busy?

JENNY: I am trying to focus more on the now. I used to never think of good things.

ANNE: What good things are you focusing on now?

JENNY: School. Completing this program. Talking more to my mother and improving my relationship with her.

ANNE: What are your best hopes for what would be different between you and your mother that would tell you that your relationship has improved?

JENNY: I think it will take time.

ANNE: What would you be doing differently when your relationship has improved with your mother?

JENNY: We would actually talk and I would be home more.

Empathizing and Addiction

Patients and families who suffer from addiction experience tremendous pain, distress, anguish, grief, and sorrow, requiring a great deal of emotional yes-set "for you" responses and compliments. Often parents or other VIPs in a patient's life feel ambivalent about forcing their loved ones into treatment. Educating patients and their VIPs on the effectiveness of treatment, whether voluntary or mandated, can provide them with much-needed reassurance (National Institute on Drug Abuse 2009). The strength, perseverance, and determination of patients and their VIPs to get themselves or their loved ones into treatment are critical to acknowledge and compliment. Asking them where they get their strength and determination from can amplify these strengths. Compliments can impart much-needed energy and stamina to both patients and their VIPS, enabling them to persevere when they are feeling exhausted and overwhelmed.

Adolescents frequently make threats when they are forced into treatment, from running away to dropping out of school or escalating their drug use. This generates desperation in their parents, as well as concern that they will lose their child. It is then important for the clinician to acknowledge their fears and the arduousness of their plight by providing many emotional yes-set "for you" responses. Complimenting loved ones and VIPs on their efforts to get their loved ones into treatment is also of great importance. Addiction is a deadly disease. Since the 1980s, drug-related deaths have more than doubled. Today, one in four deaths in the United States is attributed to alcohol, tobacco, or illicit drug use (National Institutes of Health National Institute on Drug Abuse United States 2007). The video "Beginning With Parental Strengths" illustrates the importance of complimenting parents for finding the necessary strength and steadfastness to seek addiction treatment for their children.

 Video Illustration: Beginning with parental strengths in addiction treatment (4:23)

Normalizing and Education in Addiction

Normalizing addiction as a disease and educating patients and their VIPs about this disease is a tool used by many clinicians and is also important in practicing solution-focused therapy (O'Hanlon and Weiner-Davis 1989). In treating those with addiction, several areas are of particular importance, beginning with the issue of addiction as a disease. Talking about addiction as a disease can help to minimize self-blame and empower families to work together as a team against the common enemy, the disease of addiction (White and Epston 1990). This permits patients and their VIPs both to externalize the disease of addiction and take credit for their recovery. When patients meet with success, compliments are furnished. When relapse occurs, the disease of addiction receives the blame. Explaining to patients and their VIPs that the disease of addiction commonly presents with symptoms of lying, stealing, and disregard for others in order to procure the drug of choice blames these harmful behaviors on the disease, which can help absolve patients of excessive guilt and empower them to move forward in their life. Validating how difficult these behaviors are for their VIPs, while providing education and normalization of their experience, can be a step toward helping patients' and their VIPs' relationship heal.

The disease of addiction most commonly begins during adolescence and can present with predictable patterns of behaviors (National Institute on Drug Abuse 2009). These patterns can be helpful for patients, clinicians, and their VIPs to understand. Not all people who experiment with drugs develop an addiction; many are able to stop. However, in those who do develop the disease, some predictable patterns emerge. Adolescents often begin with experimentation, leading to gradual behavioral difficulties such as decreases in attention span, low frustration tolerance, missed classes, declines in grades, increased truancy, changes in peer group, and discontinuation of extracurricular activities. The family becomes concerned. The adolescent begins to have daily highs, impaired thinking, and a loss of prior alibis. As the addiction continues, the adolescent begins to increase the amount and frequency of use, continues with school difficulties, and has a decreased ability to stop drug use. Often, disciplinary and legal difficulties increase and obsession with drug use escalates. The point at which patients seek help is variable. Some hit bottom, but for others, VIPs in their life become increasingly concerned and encourage their loved ones to get help, or they are mandated into treatment.

Educating patients and their VIPs about withdrawal symptoms, cravings, and postacute withdrawal symptoms can help to normalize these difficulties. Postacute withdrawal symptoms can include subjective symptoms of negative affect, depression, irritability, anxiety, and cravings (Koob 2000). Asking patients how they are coping with these symptoms conveys empathy with their discomfort while assisting them in moving forward with solutions that are working. Scaling how severe their cravings are from 1–10 and how well they are managing cravings from 1–10 helps to normalize these difficulties while sustaining the solution-focused conversation.

Providing parents and adolescents with education on normal brain development can be beneficial in showing empathy with the challenges they face. The brain of an adolescent is very different from the brain of a child or an adult. The neocortical and frontal lobes are not fully developed, and there is disproportionate growth of the limbic system. This stage of brain development begins during puberty and can last up to 10 years (Casey et al. 2008). Imagine the limbic lobe as the accelerator in a race car, and the frontal lobe as bicycle brakes, and you have an image of the adolescent brain. These neurological developments present further challenges for adolescents, making it even more difficult for them to stop, think, wait, and delay gratification, especially when drugs are added into the mix. Parents are required to act as what might be called "external frontal lobes" for their child, and going "limbic on limbic" with their adolescent, though not unusual, generally does little to help the child. For the parents, acting as an external part of their child's brain is a difficult job, to say the least! For the clinician, confirming the parents' need to act as a "frontal lobe," and validating the difficulty of this task, credits them with the effort they are exerting for their child. It is important, too, for the clinician to notice the times when the child is able to stop, think, wait, and delay gratification, and to amplify these positive differences.

Parents of adolescents who suffer from addiction are in much need of support and education. Their role can be exhausting, infuriating, and discouraging. Recognizing and confirming the challenges with parents provides important emotional validation. Paying attention to positive differences—times when parents are able to provide structure, follow up on limits, set clear expectations, care for their own needs, and empathize with their child's addiction and needs—is essential.

Often patients who suffer from addiction want a pill to fix their problems. This is understandable, since they have learned that drugs can be very helpful to immediately, albeit temporarily, take away uncomfortable feelings. For patients, identifying and tolerating uncomfortable feelings without using drugs requires skill as well as expertise in knowing and expressing unmet needs. Paying attention to times when patients are able to do this, amplifying the positive differences, and reframing these challenges as opportunities to learn new skills is often met with interest.

Remaining mindful of how language is spoken is paramount. Talking with patients about how they "suffer" from addiction conveys empathy. "Having" a disease is very different from "being" the disease. Declaring that a person "is" a drug addict implies that this is who the person is and always will be. The language presumes there is no hope for change. Words are powerful!

Understanding the difference between addictive behaviors and sober behaviors can provide additional useful information for the clinician, the patient, and the patient's VIPs. Sober behaviors are actions that build trust. Addictive behaviors generate a loss of trust. When patients are honest, do what they say they will do, call when they say they will call, come home when they say they will come home, clean their room, help around the house, contribute to the family needs, follow up on their plans, remain drug free, and are respectful, trust increases and is a strong indication that patients are sober. Listening for times when patients are exhibiting sober behaviors and then amplifying these positive differences can uncover much-needed successes. Scaling how satisfied patients are in maintaining their sober behaviors from 1–10, from both their own and their VIPs' perspectives, can expound details about what is working and what it will take to move forward. Scaling satisfaction can also sustain a calm and positive conversational direction in what is often a very emotionally charged area.

Solution-Focused Therapy for Those in Recovery

Individuals who are "in" recovery know what it means and how important it is for them (Betty Ford Institute Consensus Panel 2007). There is no clear definition of recovery; however, the Betty Ford Institute Consensus Panel has defined recovery from substance dependence as "a voluntarily maintained lifestyle characterized by sobriety, personal health and citizenship" (Betty Ford Institute Consensus Panel 2007). Recovery is recognized as being multidimensional, involving more than the elimination of substance use (De Leon 2000; Laudet 2007; White 2007). Sobriety is defined as abstinence from alcohol and all other nonprescribed drugs. According to the Betty Ford Institute Consensus Panel, early sobriety lasts for at least 1 month but less than 1 year; sustained sobriety lasts for at least 1 year but less than 5 years; and stable sobriety lasts for at least 5 years (Betty Ford Institute Consensus Panel 2007).

Using solution-focused therapy during times of recovery is very beneficial. Patients who are in recovery will often demonstrate an honest desire for help and begin to learn about chemical dependence as a disease. They begin an honest self-appraisal and begin to see new possibilities for their life. They begin to have more goals for themselves and their relationships and to become more aware of others. They take more responsibility for their choices and are more able to delay gratification and to think things through instead of acting impulsively. Relationships with their parents and other important people in their life improve, and trust begins to build as they are more successful in doing things they said they would do, such as following rules and meeting expectations within the family. New or old healthy interests resume, and educational interest emerges. Patients who are involved in AA continue to attend meetings, call their sponsor, and work the program, begin to address feelings and issues while sober, and are better able to tolerate painful feelings without using drugs. Physically, they begin to take care of themselves and make healthy choices. There is renewed hope and confidence in their life.

All this takes tremendous work. Acknowledging how much hard work this takes sustains an appreciative stance and allows patients to save face should they relapse. Pausing to amplify these positive signs of recovery bolsters their accomplishments. Scaling how confident they are from 1–10 that they can continue these constructive actions enriches their achievements. Scaling how things are between them and their VIPs when they are in recovery assists them in evaluating the benefits of recovery and sober behaviors on their relationships.

Solution-Focused Therapy and Relapse

Solution-focused therapy is also helpful when patients relapse. Relapse is a part of addiction (Donovan and Witkiewitz 2012; Margolis and Zweben 2011; Marlatt et al. 2012; Wanigaratne and Keaney 2011). It is normal and to be expected. This is often painful and difficult for both patients and their VIPs to understand. Normalizing relapse as part of the disease of addiction and reframing relapse as a sign of success can be very valuable. In order for relapse to occur, patients must have had some success prior to the setback. Commencing with questions exploring how they managed to stay sober, and what helped them get back on track after their relapse, maintains the solution-focused conversation. Asking patients to scale how confident they are from

1–10 in maintaining their sobriety and how confident they think their VIPs are that they could remain sober assists patients in self-appraising where they are in their recovery. Asking patients to scale how much they need to work toward their recovery, from 1–10, assesses their motivation to change. Asking patients what their longest abstinence period was, if this was different for them, if it was helpful for them, and how they accomplished this can lead the conversation toward solutions that have worked for them in the past.

Case Illustration: Remaining Solution Focused When Patients Relapse

Lois is a 33-year-old woman who was being seen for a routine outpatient appointment after she had been treated in a rehabilitation center. She had recently relapsed. This conversation illustrates how to maintain a solution-focused conversation in times of relapse.

ANNE: What's been better since we last met?

LOIS: Nothing. Things have gotten worse.

ANNE: What's different?

> *When things are not better, asking what's different helps gain understanding in a respectful way.*

LOIS: I relapsed and feel miserable.

ANNE: It sounds like things have been very difficult for you. How have you been coping with this?

LOIS: They have been difficult. I am tired of all this and the way things are going. I don't want to stay in all this misery.

ANNE: Of course, this must be difficult for you. Where do you want to stay instead of in all this misery?

LOIS: I just want to be happy. I know what I need to do. It's just a matter of doing it.

ANNE: I am impressed that you know what you need. What do you think you need to do?

LOIS: I need to be honest, do what I say I will do, and follow up with my plans.

ANNE: I can tell you have thought a lot about this. Would this be different for you to be honest and follow up with your plans?

> *Exploring and amplifying a positive difference.*

LOIS: Yes.

ANNE: How would this be different for you?

LOIS: It isn't working, what I have been doing. I'm back in rehab again. I felt miserable lying and then relapsing and going through all the same stuff again. I actually am grateful for my relapse. I want to stay clean.

ANNE: Is this different that you want to stay clean?

> *Continuing to listen for and amplify positive differences.*

LOIS: Yes.

ANNE: How is it different?

LOIS: I want my relationship with my mother to get better. I'm so tired of all this.

ANNE: Is it helpful for you that you want to stay clean?

LOIS: Yes.

ANNE: How is it helpful for you?

LOIS: I want to get on the right path to happiness.

ANNE: Wow! That's a great road to want, happiness. Suppose you were on that road to happiness, what would you be doing differently when you are on that path?

LOIS: I would be more honest, and do the next right thing. I would put more effort in.

ANNE: What else would you be doing when you are on the right path?

LOIS: I would have a better relationship with my mother. We would be spending more time together, and she would have more trust in me.

ANNE: What else would tell you that things are better between you and your mother?

LOIS: I would be honest with her. My mother is tired of my lies and really disgusted with them. She was really angry and disappointed with me. It is so hard for me to be honest with her and with all the people in my life.

ANNE: I am impressed by your desire and love for your mother, and how painful this is for you that your mother is so disappointed. How do you think it has been helpful for you to not be honest?

LOIS: Helpful?? It hasn't been helpful.

ANNE: I know this is a strange question, but usually people do find their behaviors in some ways to be helpful or they would not continue to do them. How do you think this behavior has been helpful for you?

LOIS (*pause*): It has made me feel I can control how others feel about me. I would tell them these stories of all the things I have been through and then they would think I was making progress, which really wasn't happening.

ANNE: It sounds like it is very important for you to have others see progress you are making.

LOIS: Yes, but honest progress, real progress.

ANNE: What do you mean by honest real progress?

LOIS: I would be going somewhere in my life. I would be going to a sober living house and going to college for graphic designers.

ANNE: What else would you be doing when you make honest real progress?

LOIS: I don't know (*pause*). I would be honest and my mother would be proud of me.

ANNE: Supposing 10 is you are satisfied with the honest real progress you are hoping for and 1 is the opposite, where would you say you are now?

LOIS: 5.

ANNE: Is that number going up or down?

LOIS: Up.

ANNE: What makes it not lower than a 5?

LOIS: I know what my goals are and what it will take to get there.

The conversation continues with what else makes the number not lower and what it would take to raise it by one point. As all these cases illustrate, the solution-focused techniques used with patient suffering from addiction are similar to those used with other patients. The techniques of beginning with strengths, identifying VIPs, identifying and amplifying positive differences, identifying best hopes, and asking scaling questions are used just as with other patients.

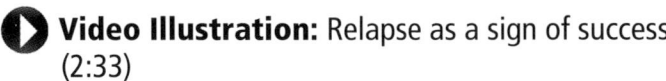 **Video Illustration:** Relapse as a sign of success (2:33)

Learning Exercise: Solution-Focused Therapy With Addiction

> Tommy was an 18-year-old man who was living with his father and step-mother. He came to his routine outpatient appointment with his father. He had been in numerous treatment facilities, including inpatient hospitals, day treatment, and rehabilitation centers, and he only recently went back to live with his parents. He was repeating his last year of high school for the second time. He initially wanted to get his GED but decided instead to go back and get a high school diploma. Tommy has struggled with substance dependence since he was 12 years old. His drugs of choice were alcohol and cannabis, but he had also used cocaine and ecstasy. Two weeks ago, to celebrate his 18th birthday, he went out with his girlfriend to get high. His father was very upset about this decision. Tommy had started summer school, which his parents had agreed to pay for. His parents had recently established several expectations for him as conditions for him to be able to stay at home with them. He needed to go to school, do his chores, help around the house, remain clean and sober, and be respectful. Tommy recently was taken off probation when he turned 18. His parents made it clear that Tommy would need to pay them back for summer school if he did not pass his summer classes. His father was also concerned because Tommy had recently stopped taking the sertraline that was prescribed to him.

Break up into groups of three to five and discuss the following:

1. What solution-focused questions would you consider asking Tommy and his father?
2. If you could ask Tommy and his father only three questions, what would you choose to ask?
3. What compliments could you give Tommy and his father based on only the information presented?
4. What are possible positive differences that could be explored?
5. What are possible scaling questions that you could ask both Tommy and his father?
6. What are some possible goal negotiation questions that could be asked of Tommy and his father?

KEY POINTS

- Especially in working with externally motivated patients, finding ways to provide genuine compliments is critical to building engagement.

- Inviting patients to talk about what they most appreciate about their VIPs accrues vital relationship deposits while strengthening bonds that have often been severely damaged by the disease of addiction.

- Rather than confronting a patient's denial, asking their "good reasons" for using drugs and "how drugs are helpful for them" respectfully explores their motivation to use drugs.

- Scaling how helpful and unhelpful drugs are, both from patients' and VIPs' perspectives, further amplifies ambivalence.

- Patients and families who suffer from addiction benefit from frequent use of "for you" responses and compliments.

- Talking about addiction as a disease can help to minimize self-blame and empower families to work together against the common enemy, the "disease of addiction."

- Scaling questions can be asked to amplify how well patients are managing their cravings, working toward their recovery, and maintaining sober behaviors.

- Scaling how well things are "between" patients and their VIPs when they are sober can assist them in evaluating the benefits of their recovery on their relationships.

- Relapse is a sign of success.

- Asking patients what has helped them get back on track and how they stayed sober prior to their relapse explores for positive differences.

References

Anderson H, Goolishian H: Thinking about multi-agency work with substance abusers and their families: a language systems approach. Journal of Strategic and Systemic Therapies 10:20–35, 1991

Berg IK: Solution-focused brief therapy with substance abusers, in Psychotherapy and Substance Abuse: A Practitioner's Handbook. Edited by Washton AM. New York, Guilford, 1996, pp 223–242

Berg IK, De Jong P: Engagement through complimenting. Journal of Family Psychotherapy 16:51–56, 2005

Berg IK, Miller SD: Working With the Problem Drinker: A Solution-Focused Approach. New York, WW Norton, 1992

Berg IK, Shafer KC: Working with mandated substance abusers: the language of solutions, in Clinical Work With Substance-Abusing Clients, 2nd Edition. Edited by Straussner SLA. New York, Guilford, 2004, pp 82–102

Betty Ford Institute Consensus Panel: What is recovery? A working definition from the Betty Ford Institute. J Subst Abuse Treat 33:221–228, 2007

Campbell J, Elder J, Gallagher D, et al: Crafting the "tap on the shoulder": a compliment template for solution-focused therapy. Am J Fam Ther 27:35–47, 1999

Casey BJ, Jones RM, Hare TA: The adolescent brain. Ann N Y Acad Sci 1124:111–126, 2008

De Leon G: The Therapeutic Community: Theory, Model, and Method. New York, Springer, 2000

de Shazer S, Isebaert L: The Bruges Model: a solution-focused approach to problem drinking. Journal of Family Psychotherapy 14:43–52, 2004

Donovan D, Witkiewitz K: Relapse prevention: from radical idea to common practice. Addict Res Theory 20:204–217, 2012

Koob GF: Neurobiology of addiction. Toward the development of new therapies. Ann N Y Acad Sci 909:170–185, 2000

Laudet AB: What does recovery mean to you? Lessons from the recovery experience for research and practice. J Subst Abuse Treat 33:243–256, 2007

Margolis RD, Zweben JE: Relapse prevention, in Treating Patients With Alcohol and Other Drug Problems: An Integrated Approach, 2nd Edition. Washington, DC, American Psychological Association, 2011, pp 199–224

Marlatt GA, Bowen S, Lustyk MKB: Substance abuse and relapse prevention, in Wisdom and Compassion in Psychotherapy: Deepening Mindfulness in Clinical Practice. Edited by Germer CK, Siegel RD. New York, Guilford, 2012, pp 221–233

McCollum EE, Trepper TS: Family Solutions for Substance Abuse: Clinical and Counseling Approaches. Binghamton, NY, Haworth, 2001

Minkoff K: Developing standards of care for individuals with co-occurring psychiatric and substance use disorders. Psychiatr Serv 52:597–599, 2001

National Institutes of Health National Institute on Drug Abuse United States: Drugs, Brains, and Behavior: The Science of Addiction. 2007. Available at: http://www.drugabuse.gov/publications/science-addiction. Accessed February 23, 2013.

National Institute on Drug Abuse: Principles of Drug Addiction Treatment: A Research-Based Guide, 2nd Edition (NIH Publ No 09-4180). Bethesda, MD, National Institute on Drug Abuse, 2009

O'Hanlon WH, Weiner-Davis M: In Search of Solutions: A New Direction in Psychotherapy. New York, WW Norton, 1989

Pichot T: Co-creating solutions for substance abuse. Journal of Systemic Therapies 20:1–23, 2001

Pichot T, Smock SA: Solution-Focused Substance Abuse Treatment. New York, Routledge/Taylor & Francis Group, 2009

Wanigaratne S, Keaney F: Relapse prevention for the 21st century, in Principles and Practice of Group Work in Addictions. Edited by Hill R, Harris J. New York, Routledge/Taylor & Francis Group, 2011, pp 30–44

White WL: Addiction recovery: its definition and conceptual boundaries. J Subst Abuse Treat 33:229–241, 2007

White M, Epston D: Narrative Means to Therapeutic Ends. New York, WW Norton, 1990

Yeager KR, Gregoire TK: Crisis intervention application of brief solution-focused therapy in addictions, in Crisis Intervention Handbook: Assessment, Treatment, and Research, 3rd Edition. Edited by Roberts AR. New York, Oxford University Press, 2005, pp 566–601

CHAPTER 11

Solution-Focused Supervision

In recent years it has become increasingly important for clinicians to collaborate with systems of caregivers, act as consultants to agencies, and provide a supervisory role. This is particularly true for child and adolescent psychiatrists, who often are working with multiple systems including parents, schools, community centers, residential treatment centers, other health care and mental health providers, religious institutions, primary health care providers, child welfare agencies, juvenile justice systems, programs for those with developmental disabilities, early childhood programs, and substance abuse services (Chenven 2010; Sarvet and Wegner 2010; Winters et al. 2007). Solution-focused conversational skills can be extremely valuable in roles such as working as a consultant with staff and agencies, facilitating team meetings with multiple providers, and providing supervision. This chapter will attempt to provide a guide as to how to best accomplish these challenging jobs.

Solution-Focused Assumptions in Supervision

When a clinician is required to work as a consultant with a team, provide training for staff, or act in a supervisory role, certain solution-focused working assumptions apply (Table 11–1). These assumptions were described by Insoo Kim Berg (1994).

Clinical supervision and consultation play essential roles in education, training, and clinical care, yet they are probably the least investigated, discussed, and developed aspects of clinical teaching (Kilminster and Jolly 2000). Supervision and consultation are complex activities that occur in a variety of settings, and most importantly, involve interpersonal exchanges.

TABLE 11–1.   Solution-focused assumptions to make when working in the supervisory role

Unless the contrary is proven, we believe the following:

- Everybody wants to do a good job.
- All workers want to be proud of their work.
- All workers want to make a difference.
- Everybody has reasonable problem-solving skills. Our task is to add on solution-building skills.
- An important responsibility of the supervisor is to help the supervisee/staff identify and enhance their solution-building resources.
- When staff/supervisee feels respected by their supervisor/superior they will in turn deal with their patients in a respectful manner.

In most definitions, supervision entails promoting professional development and ensuring patient safety, and it is usually understood as partly hierarchical and evaluative (Kilminster and Jolly 2000). Kilminster and Jolly define supervision as "the provision of monitoring, guidance and feedback on matters of personal, professional and educational development in the context of the doctor's care of patients. This would include the ability to anticipate a doctor's strengths and weaknesses, in particular clinical situations in order to maximize patient safety" (Kilminster and Jolly 2000, p. 828). The ultimate purpose of supervision and consultation is to improve the patient's outcome and experience. Therefore, improvements in outcomes for patients are one major test of effective supervision and consultation.

Supervision and consultation involve addressing the supervisee's needs, the patient's needs, and the agency's needs. The supervisor relationship also involves both hierarchical and evaluative components, adding further complexity to the task of supervision. Supervision and consultation involve simultaneously addressing all these requirements while maintaining a positive relationship with the supervisee.

Solution-focused supervision approaches are designed to construct a sense of competence and confidence with the supervisee and agency or staff, respectively (Briggs and Miller 2005). Just as solution-focused therapists position themselves to be in a state of being informed by the patient, solution-focused supervisors position themselves in a state of being informed by the supervisee (Briggs and Miller 2005).

Learning solution-focused supervision allows a supervisor to have a twofold effect (Trenhaile 2005). The first effect is to enhance a clinician's, agency's, or staff's sense of themselves as competent and successful professionals. The second is to indirectly influence patient outcome through the supervisory or consulting relationship. This approach is empowering to the supervisee, the supervisor, and the patient (Trenhaile 2005).

Briggs and Miller identify strategies and practices that enhance how supervisors can assist therapists in building, augmenting, extending, and accentuating the therapist's clinical strengths, skills, and successes (Briggs and Miller 2005). Solution-focused supervision involves recognizing and amplifying successes and competencies, rather than accentuating deficits (O'Hanlon and Weiner Davis 1989; Thomas 1994; Trepper et al. 2006). Solution-focused supervision seeks to set up a cooperative, goal-oriented relationship that assumes the supervisee possesses the strength, resources, and ability to resolve a complaint and achieve training goals (Thomas 1994). Trenhaile states that the primary focus of a solution-focused approach to mental health supervision should be patient outcome, with mental health worker development as a secondary result (Trenhaile 2005). Trenhaile suggests a four-part format for solution-focused supervision: 1) establish an atmosphere of competence, 2) search for patient-based solutions, 3) provide feedback to the supervisee, and 4) provide follow-up supervision (Trenhaile 2005). Briggs and Miller (2005) talk about how success-enhancing supervisors guide the therapist toward recognizing his or her successes, building a sense of competency. Constructing a supervisory relationship wherein the therapist is able to confidently approach and conduct sessions with an undistracted focus on the patient will also allow therapists to do a better job of serving their patients (Briggs and Miller 2005).

Practicing solution-focused supervision does not mean forcing this model onto the supervisees. Just as proponents of solution-focused therapy believe there is no single way to solve problems, there is no single best way to do therapy. When supervisors become too focused on their own goal of forcing a particular way of therapy onto the supervisee, often opportunities to learn from their supervisee are missed. Thomas proposes that supervisors tend to adopt one of three positions: the "guru" imparts expert knowledge on practice that supervisees seek to copy, the "gatekeeper" arbitrates whether supervisees will belong to the community of practitioners, and the "guide" collaborates with supervisees to foster learning that will elicit their unique version of practice (Thomas 1994). Solution-focused supervision relates well to the "guide" position through the process of asking carefully constructed questions.

Three Phases of Solution-Focused Supervision

Solution-focused supervision can be separated into three phases. The initial phase focuses on the supervisee's strengths and goals rather than on problems and mistakes (Wetchler 1990). The second phase centers on patient-focused supervision (Trenhaile 2005). Patient-focused supervision addresses the needs and goals of the patient, using solution-focused approaches with the supervisee. The third phase focuses on supervisee feedback, including compliments, education, and possible homework assignments. This three-phase approach to supervision attends to the simultaneous needs of the supervisee, patient, and supervisor, all of which are essential for effective supervision and consultation.

Phase 1A: Identifying Supervisee's Strengths and Resources

Just as a solution-focused interview begins with an exploration of strengths and competencies with patients, solution-focused supervision begins with an exploration of strengths and competencies with the supervisee. Commencing solution-focused supervision is similar to beginning a solution-focused interview. Both begin by asking about strengths and resources. Just as when patients are asked about what they are good at and enjoy, supervisees are asked what skills and strategies they have found most effective when working with their patients. This is followed by asking what else they have found helpful and how they have accomplished this. Often supervisees talk about showing empathy, listening, and understanding. These words and the supervisee's exact language can be examined in more detail by asking what supervisees "do" with their patient when they are showing empathy, listening, and understanding, and asking what they mean by these words. Using the supervisees' exact words and exploring their language is practiced in the same way as with patients and likewise promotes engagement and a collaborative working relationship with the supervisee. Peter De Jong invites supervisees to share success stories they have experienced when working with patients and explores with the supervisees ways large or small in which they incorporated solution-focused practice into work with their patients (Nelson 2005). Table 11–2 shows questions to commence with in working with a supervisee. The purpose of these questions is to initiate the supervisor/supervisee relationship by identifying and uncovering strengths and resources of the supervisee.

Just as in working with patients and identifying their VIPs (very important people), it is essential to ask supervisees who are the most important people in their work system who would tell them they are being successful and doing a good job. Terri Pichot and colleagues describe how to reorient the sense of who the patient is so that it includes the patient's system, and in so doing remains faithful to the solution-focused belief that there is only a problem if the patient or anyone in the patient's system views it as such (Pichot and Dolan 2003; Pichot and Smock 2009). Just as each patient has his or her own unique system, supervisees also have their own unique sys-

TABLE 11–2. Beginning with supervisee's strengths and resources

- What skills and strategies have you found most helpful in working with patients?
- What else have you found most helpful in working with patients?
- What would your patients say you have done that has been most helpful for them?
- What else would your patients say you have done that has been helpful for them?
- What have been the most helpful training experiences for you?
- What have you learned from your patients that has been most helpful for you in providing effective treatment?
- What kinds of supervision have been most helpful for you?
- What interests and life experiences have been most helpful for you in working with your patients?
- With which types of problems, people, situations, or families have you had most success in helping?
- What have you tried in therapy with your patients that has been most helpful for your patients?
- How has your therapy and work improved since you started training?
- What are you doing differently that has been helpful since you started your training?
- When do you feel the most competent and successful with patients?
- What successes have you experienced this week with your patients?
- What successful interactions have you experienced with patients?
- What successful interventions have you experienced with patients?
- What successful outcomes have you experienced with patients?
- Think about times you felt lacking in the right skills or overwhelmed with your work, how have you managed?
- What has kept you going?
- Where did you get the strength and courage to continue on with your work?
- What do you need to keep doing to keep these successful activities going?

tems in which they work, based on their unique circumstances. Supervisees' VIP lists will of course include their patients and their patients' VIPs. Supervisees' VIPs may also include the agency staff they work with as well as their supervisor, colleagues, training director, administrative staff, other therapists involved with the care of their patients, DCF workers, and teachers. A supervisee's system may also include agency policies, legal mandates, and mandatory reporting requirements. Although these aspects of the supervisee's system are not people, they are included in this list of VIPs because these are requirements that supervisees must attend to in order to be successful in their job. Asking supervisees whether they are knowledgeable about agency policies and requirements that will help them be successful, such as completing notes in a timely manner, responding to calls and emergencies, and fulfilling mandatory reporting requirements respectfully educates supervisees about how they will be evaluated, helping them identify the unique VIPs that are essential for them to know in order to be successful in their job. The questions listed in Table 11–3 are helpful in assessing VIPs with supervisees during the initial phase of supervision.

TABLE 11–3.   Questions that identify the supervisee's VIPs

- Who are the VIPs (patients/treatment providers/supervisor/agency) most important for you that would tell you that you are doing a good job and being successful?

- Who else?

- What would these VIPs say you have done so far that has been most helpful for them?

- What would these VIPs say you are doing that would tell them you are doing a good job?

- What else would they say you are doing that tells them you are helpful and doing a good job?

- What would your VIPs (patient/agency/training director/treatment team/ supervisor) say is necessary to tell them you are doing a good job and meeting their requirements?

- On a scale of 1–10, how helpful do you suppose your VIPs (patient/family/ treatment team/agency/supervisor) would say you have been to your patient?

- On a scale of 1–10, how satisfied do you suppose your VIPs (agency/supervisor) are that you have met their requirements (such as completing notes, following up with phone calls, and collaborating with staff)?

 Video Illustration: Supervision: beginning with successes (3:17)

Case Illustration: Beginning With Successes

Sandy was a new child psychiatry fellow. She had just completed 3 years of adult psychiatry training, and this was her first day starting her child psychiatry outpatient rotation. She was both anxious and excited about starting to see children and had been eagerly awaiting starting her fellowship. The following is the initial supervision meeting with Sandy. She had just seen the first child patient of her training experience. Notice that I start with identifying and amplifying her strengths and competencies. This is followed by asking what has been most helpful in her training, much like asking patients what has been most helpful in their treatment thus far. Goal negotiation, through exploration of her best hopes for her training experience, follows as the next step.

ANNE: So, you made it through your first patient—congratulations. How did it go?

I commence the interview by complimenting her on getting through her first patient encounter.

SANDY: It went pretty well.

ANNE: What went pretty well?

SANDY: She seems to be doing well and seemed to be comfortable talking with me.

ANNE: What do you think you did to help her feel comfortable?

SANDY: I asked some of the questions that we talked about today.

ANNE: What questions seemed to help her feel more comfortable?

This question helps her to reflect and to notice what questions were most helpful for her patient.

SANDY: Starting off with what she was good at and asking her mother what has been most helpful so far in her treatment. It was nice to finally start seeing kids. I've been waiting a long time in my training to see kids.

ANNE: I'm sure. Training is a long haul. You have worked a long time to get here. I am wondering what training and life experiences have been most helpful for you?

SANDY: I think I do best with hands-on experience and I really try to focus on evidence-based practices.

ANNE: What do you mean by hands-on practice?

SANDY: Being able to see enough patients and watching what others do. I want to get as much experience as I can.

ANNE: What other training and life experiences have been most helpful for you?

I explore further details about helpful training experiences for her. This will help me know what kinds of learning are most helpful for her.

SANDY: During medical school, I researched child psychiatry and realized the incredible shortage of and need for child psychiatrists, especially in the state that I come from. I really want to go back there and try to make a difference.

ANNE: I am impressed that you sought out this detailed information, and how committed you are to making a difference. What else have you found helpful in your training and life experience?

SANDY: My adult training was helpful, especially my training in intellectual disabilities.

ANNE: How was training in intellectual disabilities helpful for you?

SANDY: It felt a lot like helping kids. I had to gather information from many sources and understand the whole system.

ANNE: I am impressed with all the skills you have already gained. What else was helpful about that experience?

SANDY: I needed to be attentive to small changes.

ANNE: Is that something you are good at, paying attention to small changes?

I continue to listen for strengths throughout the conversation, taking these opportunities to compliment her.

SANDY: Yes, I think I'm a pretty good listener.

ANNE: That's a great skill to have. What do you do that tells you that you are good listener?

SANDY: I am a pretty quiet person and don't interrupt people. I think that helps people feel like I am listening to them.

ANNE: Has that been helpful for you?

SANDY: Yes.

ANNE: How has that been helpful for you?

SANDY: I think it helps patients feel comfortable with me and helps them to trust me.

ANNE: Being a good listener is such a critical skill in this field. It's great you have this ability. What areas do you feel most confident about in your training?

This question helps to uncover additional strengths and capabilities.

SANDY: I think I am pretty good at making people comfortable.

ANNE: What else do you feel most confident about?

SANDY: I'm soft spoken and don't interrupt.

ANNE: What do you mean soft spoken?

SANDY: My tone of voice. I think it's my Southern hospitality. It's been hard sometimes adjusting to the culture here. It's so different from where I come from.

ANNE: Of course, that must be difficult for you adjusting to this culture. How did you manage?

SANDY: I think it was just exposure, and realizing this is the way people are here. At first I thought people were criticizing me. Then I learned it was just a different culture. It was tough getting used to some of the supervisors.

ANNE: I am impressed by how you coped with this. Of all your training experience, what supervision has been most helpful for you?

This question helps us learn together what kinds of supervision will be most helpful for her.

SANDY: Dr. S. He was really helpful.

ANNE: What did he do that was most helpful for you?

SANDY: He was very engaging and interactive. He would do a lot of teaching in our meetings.

ANNE: What teaching was most helpful for you?

SANDY: He would give examples of his own practice and was always nice and respectful.

ANNE: Who else has been most helpful in your training?

SANDY: Dr. W.

ANNE: What did she do that was helpful for you?

SANDY: She was positive and nice and always seemed interested in my well-being. She was so supportive.

ANNE: What do you think she did that helped you feel supported?

SANDY: She would never tell me this is the way to do it. She would say things like, "One way you might consider doing this is so-and-so."

ANNE: What else did she do that was helpful?

SANDY: If I asked her a question, she would always go to the evidence and we would talk about it. She was always available and seemed really interested in patient care.

ANNE: Were there training experiences that were not helpful for you?

SANDY: When supervisors were critical. There was one supervisor early on in my training who would only point out what I was doing wrong and who was really focused on only her way of doing things. I think it made it especially hard because I had so little experience.

Phase 1B: Goal Negotiation With the Supervisee

Following the exploration of strengths and VIPs, the supervisor negotiates goals with the supervisee. This order of questioning mirrors that of patients—the only change being the focus on the supervisees and their best hopes for their training and supervision. Table 11–4 presents a list of goal-setting questions to ask supervisees.

TABLE 11–4. Goal negotiation questions with the supervisee

- What are your [the supervisee's] best hopes for supervision that would tell you it was helpful for you and not a waste of time?
- What else are your best hopes for supervision?
- Suppose 10 is you are confident in your skills and 1 is the opposite, what number would you say you are at now?
- What number makes it not lower?
- What else makes it not lower?
- What would it take to raise it by one point?
- What would you like to accomplish in the next hour so this meeting is useful for you?
- Suppose 10 is you are satisfied with the progress toward your goals, and 1 is the opposite, where would you say you are now?
- What makes it not lower?
- What else makes it not lower?
- What would it take to raise it one point?

Case Illustration: Goal Negotiation With Supervisees

ANNE: What are your best hopes for your training so you can say it has been helpful for you and worth all this time and hard work?

SANDY: I want to learn the evidence base. I know there isn't that much, but I want to know this.

ANNE: Of course, that is so important. What else would tell you that your training has been helpful for you?

SANDY: That I learn to interact with children and families in a nonjudgmental way, but still get a comprehensive treatment plan.

ANNE: What else would be important for you?

SANDY: That I keep my medical foundation and get as many perspectives as I can. I know that particularly in psychiatry there are many different approaches. I want to know why and the rationale for these approaches.

ANNE: I can tell you have thought a lot about this. What skills do you think you need to have when you have completed your training that would tell you that you are satisfied with your training?

SANDY: I think I'm interested in an academic component. I helped develop a training component in my adult residency and really like to teach.

Notice that through this process of goal negotiation, additional strengths are revealed; these are important to amplify.

ANNE: Tell me about this training component you developed.

SANDY: I needed to help new interns show that they are ready to see patients.

ANNE: Wow, that sounds very challenging! How did you do this?

SANDY: I had to develop a PowerPoint presentation and create pre- and post-test scenarios to demonstrate that residents could be able to ask for help.

ANNE: How did you do this?

SANDY: I had to teach and evaluate the residents on whether things are urgent, emergent, or in need of a timely intervention. I ended up presenting this at a conference.

ANNE: That's fantastic. You have a lot of skill with teaching.

SANDY: I think I may be interested in becoming a training director or having some teaching component to my training.

ANNE: That's great. I am impressed with all the skills that you have, your passion, and the wonderful goals you have. My hope is that I will be able to assist you in meeting these goals.

This conversation illustrates how to incorporate solution-focused approaches within the initial supervisory meeting. The conversation began with finding strengths and giving compliments, amplifying positive differences, and beginning an exploration of her goals. In this way, it is similar to beginning a conversation with a patient. Many strengths and talents were uncovered, including training experiences and supervisors that have been helpful for her. This dialog set up a collaborative relationship as well as accumulating deposits that will help to facilitate engagement and a positive working relationship.

Phase 2: Patient-Focused Supervision

After enough time has been spent with the supervisee exploring his or her strengths, VIPs, and goals, it is time to proceed to the second phase, patient-focused supervision. This phase involves a case presentation and a search for patient-based solutions (Trenhaile 2005). Patient-focused supervision focuses on the goals and needs of the patient, using solution-focused techniques. The time to proceed to this phase of supervision is variable depending on the individual needs of the supervisee. Supervisees who feel anxious, uncertain, or overwhelmed will require more emotional yes-set responses and compliments prior to this phase. When supervisees are just starting their training and are treating patients for the first time or experiencing very challenging cases, it is critical to spend enough time validating how challenging these situations are "for them." Making statements such as "I can see how hard you are working for your patient," or "I appreciate how much thought you put into this situation for your patient" are examples of providing emotional validation for the supervisee. Asking supervisees how they are coping and handling these difficult situations and what they need orients the conversation toward what they are already doing to manage these demanding circumstances, conveying their capabilities. Listening for opportunities to compliment supervisees on their work when they are presenting their cases, just as when patients are telling their stories, is essential in order to uncover and amplify the successes they are already achieving. Asking supervisees what they have tried that has been most helpful for their patients or what they are doing that is working for their patients can assist the supervisor in uncovering successes that supervisees are already attaining. Asking what else they have tried that is helpful for the client digs for more details of their successes. Just as with patients, it is critical to listen for opportunities to compliment the supervisee and identify positive differences within the dialog, providing plenty of deposits early on and throughout the conversation. Likewise, it is important to amplify these compliments and positive differences using the same line of questions that are asked of patients to amplify their positive differences. Each person requires differing amounts of deposits depending on his or her reaction. Just as in work with patients, supervisees will let you know if they need more emotional yes-set responses and compliments. Increased defensiveness, lack of cooperation, and increased anxiety may all be indications the supervisor is moving faster than the supervisee is comfortable with.

As noted, patient-focused supervision involves a case presentation and a search for patient-based solutions, helping the supervisee concretely focus on the patient's strengths, needs, goals, and successes (Trenhaile 2005). The questions asked of the supervisee mirror the questions that are asked in a solution-focused interview, and in this way they maintain the supervisory focus on the patient's needs. The first questions asked of a supervisee in the patient-based portion of supervision are directed toward what "your patient" would say are the supervisee's strengths, resources, and VIPs. Incorporating the words "what your patient would say" within questions posed to the supervisee respectfully maintains the focus on the patient while helping the supervisee reflect on these questions. Supervision is a process that is once removed from the patient. Asking supervisees what "your patient would say" is a linguistic technique that addresses how to maintain the focus on the patient when the patient is not directly involved in the supervisory process. When supervisees are able to answer these questions, it provides opportunities to explore whether they thought these questions were helpful for the patient, as well as opportunities to amplify the supervisee's skills. Asking the supervisee what "your patient" would say are his or her best hopes for treatment, what "your patient" wants help with, what "your patient" has tried that has been helpful for him or her, who "your patient" would say are his or her VIPs, and what "your patient" most appreciates about these VIPs all assist the supervisee in learning solution-focused skills while maintaining the focus on the patient. Asking the supervisee how "your patient" describes a 10-rated or miracle day, what "your patient" would say he or she would be doing differently when things are a 10, what "your patient" would say would be different between the patient and VIPs at a rating of 10, where "your patient" would rate his or her satisfaction with how things are going now on a scale of 1–10, how "your patient" would rate how he or she is coping and where his or her strength comes from—these questions all maintain the supervisory focus on the needs of the patient while simultaneously teaching supervisees the important questions to focus on with their patients. Table 11–5 lists questions used with supervisees during the patient-focused portion of supervision.

The search for patient-based solutions also involves asking supervisees what they think their patient would say the therapist is doing that is most helpful for the patient. This question assists supervisees in thinking about ways they are being useful from the patient's perspective. Asking supervisees to reflect on what "your patient" would say the therapist is doing that is most helpful, asking them to rate how helpful they think "your patient" would rate them from 1–10, what makes the number not lower, and what it would take to raise it by one point aids supervisees in gaining perspective on their helpfulness from the patient's perspective. Asking supervisees to rate how "your patient" would rate things "between" them from 1–10 assists in the evaluation of the strength of their relationship and treatment engagement. Asking supervisees to rate how confident "your patient" is that treatment will be successful assesses how optimistically the supervisee views treatment. Table 11–6 displays questions that explore treatment effectiveness with supervisees from the patient's perspective.

▶ **Video Illustration:** Patient-focused supervision (4:32)

TABLE 11–5. **Questions to ask the supervisee during patient-focused supervision**

- What would "your patient" say she (he) is good at and enjoys?
- What else would she say?
- Who would "your patient" say her VIPs are?
- What would "your patient say" she appreciates most about her VIPs?
- What else would she say she appreciates about her VIPs?
- What would "your patient" say are her best hopes for treatment?
- What would "your patient" say she has tried that has been most helpful for her?
- What does "your patient" want help with that would tell her meeting with you is worthwhile?
- What would "your patient" say she would be doing differently when she is meeting her goals?
- What else would she say she is doing differently?
- What would "your patient" say her VIPs would notice when she is getting the help she needs?
- What would "your patient" say her miracle 10 day would look like?
- What would "your patient" say she would be doing when she is at a 10?
- What else would she say she is doing?
- What would she say her VIPs would notice her doing when it is a 10 day?
- Where would she say she is now on a scale of 1–10?
- What would she say is the reason it is not lower?
- What would she say it would take to raise it by one point?
- Where would "your patient" rate her progress with treatment on a scale of 1–10?
- What number would "your patient" say she needs to be at in order to end treatment?
- How helpful would "your patient" say her medications are from 1–10?
- What would "your patient" say are her best hopes for a medication?

Phase 3: Feedback, Education, and Homework

The next phase of supervision involves feedback to the supervisee (Trenhaile 2005). The feedback includes giving compliments, summarizing and enumerating the positive differences identified within the conversation, providing education for the supervisee, and confirming and negotiating the supervisee's goals. Compliments reinforce and enhance supervisees' strengths, resources, and successes. Listing the positive differences and successes that have been uncovered further amplifies their successes. Ask-

TABLE 11–6.   Questions that explore treatment effectiveness with supervisees from the patient's perspective

- What would "your patient" say you have done that has been most helpful so far?
- What else would he (she) say you have done that has been helpful?
- Supposing 10 is "your patient" is satisfied with his treatment with you and 1 is the opposite, what number do you think he would rate treatment?
- What makes it not lower?
- What would make it one point higher?
- What do you suppose "your patient" would say you are doing that is most helpful for him?
- Is this different for you?
- How is it different for you?
- Was it helpful to do this?
- How was it helpful to do this?
- How did you do it?
- How else did you do it?
- How helpful do you suppose "your patient" would say you are on a scale of 1–10?
- What makes the number not lower?
- What would it take to make it one point higher?
- Where do you suppose "your patient" would rate your relationship on a scale of 1–10?
- What makes it not lower?
- What would "your patient" say would make it one point higher?
- How confident are you on a scale of 1–10 that you can help your patient achieve his goals?
- Is this number going up or down?
- What makes it not lower?
- What would it take to raise your confidence by one point?

ing if there is any other information they feel would be helpful to discuss opens the discussion for any further help they need.

There are times when supervisees may be in need of education. One way to offer education is to invite them to consider whether the information you were planning on sharing with them would be helpful for them, maintaining a nonassuming stance within the conversation. Usually supervisees appreciate the information given. Asking supervisees to do more of what's working with their patients, to pay attention to when the patient's scale goes up one point, and to pay attention to when things are working with the patients are all possible homework tasks to assign to supervisees. Homework tasks can also be framed as a challenge for supervisees: to try a new question, to pay attention to useful questions and techniques that are helpful for their clients, or to try some scaling questions.

Follow-up supervision involves the same process as follow-up sessions with patients. Follow-up supervision begins by asking supervisees what they found helpful, what worked with patients, and what interactions they had success with since the last meeting. These questions can uncover positive differences that can then be amplified. Asking supervisees what "your patient" would say is better or different maintains the focus of supervision on the patient. Scaling how well things are going with a particular patient, what makes the rating not lower, and what would make it one point higher further amplifies successes and goals. If things are worse, bridging both compliments and emotional yes-set responses to supervisees with questions about how they are coping, what they have tried to do to help their patient, and what "your patient" would notice that would tell the patient that things are getting better, are possible ways to help supervisees in these challenging situations. The case below illustrates a follow-up session with a supervisee.

Case Illustration: Follow-Up Supervision

Tom was treating a 6-year-old girl who was struggling with anxiety and irritability. He was concerned about whether he should have contacted protective services about this child and was anxious about whether he had done the right thing. The following is an excerpt from this conversation.

ANNE: How could I be most helpful for you today so this meeting is useful for you?

TOM: My 6-year-old patient came in with her mother and sister. She is a talented little girl but has been through a lot. Her parents divorced and she witnessed domestic violence between her parents. Her mother can present as very irritable and doesn't have much frustration tolerance. Today, her mother revealed that she hit her daughter after she found out she stole a bracelet from her teenage sister. I was very upset when I heard this and wasn't sure what to do.

ANNE: This must have been very upsetting for you. How did you handle this situation?

TOM: I first listened and then asked her mother how she coped with this.

ANNE: Was it helpful to ask her mother this?

One way to amplify this success and encourage the supervisee to reflect on his interventions is to ask him if he thought this was helpful for the patient. This maintains the conversation on the patient, while providing an indirect compliment to the supervisee.

TOM: It was because she then started talking about how when she hit her child, she noticed that it didn't help. She talked about seeing her own sister handle her children differently and wanting to do things differently with her own child.

ANNE: Was this different that "she noticed" her sister handling things differently with her own children?

I amplify this potential positive difference in the same way as with patients, beginning the query by asking how he did it, was it helpful, how it was helpful, was it different, and how it was different. These questions create a conversation in which the supervisee talks about what is working for the patient, increasing his sense of self-efficacy as a clinician, while simultaneously maintaining the focus of supervision on what is working for the patient. Notice that I am using the exact language of the supervisee.

TOM: Yes.

ANNE: How was this different for her?

TOM: I don't think she had noticed this before. She would yell and hit her daughter, and all this would do would be make her daughter shut down and go into her shell. It wasn't working.

ANNE: What did "she notice" differently that her sister did with her own children?

Asking the supervisee to reflect on what his patient's mother noticed was different assists him in metaphorically growing a "third ear" (noticing positive differences).

TOM: She noticed that her sister tries to talk with her children and takes time to understand them.

ANNE: What else did "she notice" about her sister's interactions with her children that you think was helpful for her?

TOM: That her sister is able to keep calm and respond to her children with questions instead of just yelling at them.

ANNE: I am impressed with how much you are noticing and listening to your patient. Was this helpful for her to notice this difference?

Weaving meaningful compliments to the supervisee throughout the conversation and asking questions that assist him in noticing positive differences concentrates the supervisee's attention on what he is doing that is helpful for their patient.

TOM: Yes, it was different.

ANNE: How was it different for her?

TOM: She said that she realized hitting her daughter wasn't working and recognized that she needed to do something differently.

ANNE: Wow! She is paying attention and really trying to make things better for her daughter. What do you think "she would say" in terms of how she did this?

TOM: I think she would say that things were not working with her daughter, and that she saw things worked better the way her sister did things.

ANNE: Did "she notice anything different between" her and her daughter when she tried to do things the way her sister did?

TOM: Yes. She said that her daughter talked more and opened up to her. I'm just concerned about whether I should report this to DCF [the state's Department of Children and Families]. Her mother can be so harsh, and I don't know if this is something I need to report on.

ANNE: These are very difficult situations. It sounds like you thought a lot about this. What do you think needs to happen?

Bridging a "for you" response and a compliment with a question focusing on what the supervisee thinks needs to happen conveys my belief that he has thought about this. It is important to explore the supervisee's ideas prior to offering suggestions.

TOM: Well, I actually called DCF and asked them whether they thought I should report on this.

ANNE: Wow! That was great you took the initiative to do this. Was it helpful to call DCF?

TOM: It was. They asked me if she had any marks, and I told them no. I explained what I told you, and they thought it would be screened out and not investigated. I'm just concerned that I do everything I can to make sure her mother doesn't beat her child.

ANNE: Of course, these are some of the most difficult situations to deal with. What do you mean by doing everything you can to make sure her mother does not beat her child?

I explore what he means by "doing everything," using his exact words, just as I would do with patients.

TOM: I just want to make sure she is safe, but I also don't want to ruin my relationship with her mother so she won't come back. They both really need treatment and I don't want to jeopardize my relationship with them.

ANNE: These are such challenging situations for all of us. I can tell you have thought a lot about this. What have you tried to do to evaluate her safety?

TOM: I talked to her mother about my legal obligation, that I am a mandatory reporter and that if I'm concerned about her daughter's safety I will need to report my concerns.

ANNE: Wow! You did a lot. That must have been difficult for you. Was it helpful?

TOM: I think so. She didn't seem surprised by this.

ANNE: What else did you try?

TOM: I'm not sure what else to do.

This process of questioning eventually led the supervisee to let me know he didn't know what else to do, indicating his need of further education.

ANNE: Would it be helpful for you to hear how I evaluate safety in these very difficult situations?

Offering education in the form of a question confirms whether this would be useful for him.

TOM: Yes, it would be very helpful.

Confirmation is obtained.

ANNE: The first thing that I do is to provide emotional yes-set responses to both the mother and her daughter. For example, I might say to the mother that this must have been very difficult "for you" to find out your daughter stole a bracelet, and it must be very difficult "for you" to stay calm and manage this situation. I would also provide emotional yes-set responses to her daughter. For example, it must have been very difficult "for you" to get hit by your mother and it must really stink "for you" that you got into trouble like this. In this way, I am providing emotional yes-set responses to both of them prior to proceeding with questions. I have found that this can help them both feel validated, while modeling for her mother how to empathize with her child. You noticed many positive differences about the mother, such as her ability to notice how her sister's style of interaction with her children was more helpful, her honesty and openness to try something different to be helpful for her daughter, and her willingness to get help and do whatever is needed for her daughter. You also noticed many strengths in her daughter. I have found it very helpful to provide compliments to both the parent and the child, providing them with conversational deposits and "anesthesia" during these painful experiences. Given the concerns you have talked about, it can be very helpful to interview the mother and daughter separately, to evaluate both of their needs and concerns without the emotional intensity of them both together. Scaling questions can be particularly helpful in these situations.

TOM: What scaling questions would you ask?

ANNE: There are many possibilities. You might ask the mother how helpful it was for her to remain calm and talk with her daughter on a scale of 1–10. You might also ask how helpful it was to hit her child on a scale of 1–10. These help to amplify the mother's ambivalence. Scaling questions can also be very useful in evaluating safety. One way to evaluate safety is to ask the mother on a scale of 1–10, where 10 is she is confident that she has the skills to stay calm and talk with her daughter instead of hitting her, and 1 is the opposite, where would she say she is? This could be followed with what makes it not lower, what would it take to make it one point higher? Scaling questions can also be asked to her daughter. For example, suppose 10 is you feel safe with your mother and 1 is the opposite, where would you say you are now? What makes it not lower? What would it take to raise it one point? You might also incorporate their VIPs into these scaling questions. For example, asking her mother how confident her daughter would say she is that her mother can remain calm and not hit her on a scale of 1–10?

This illustration demonstrates how supervision involves balancing the needs of the supervisee, the needs of the patient, and the needs of the agency and reporting requirements. The supervisor was able to pay attention to the skills of the supervisee, such as that the supervisee was able to notice positive differences with his patient's mother and that he managed this difficult situation in many positive ways. It also illustrates how to incorporate educational components within the process, while maintaining the focus on the patient.

LEARNING EXERCISE: SHARING SUCCESS STORIES

Talk with a colleague and share successful interactions you have both had with patients this past week. Think about the piece of work this past year that you are most proud of, and share this with a colleague. What did you do that was most helpful for your patient? Did you do something differently? How did you know that this was helpful for your patient? What do you think your patient would say you did that was most helpful for him or her? How did you accomplish this? Are there any further questions or ideas that have been generated as a result of talking about this success with someone? Take some time to reflect with each other on what it was like to share success stories with each other. Was it helpful, and if so, how?

KEY POINTS

- Solution-focused supervision allows a supervisor to have a twofold effect: to enhance a clinician's sense of competency and to indirectly influence patient outcome through the supervisory relationship.

- Solution-focused supervision seeks to set up a collaborative, goal-oriented relationship that assumes the supervisee possesses the resources and skills needed to achieve training goals.

- Solution-focused supervision can be separated into three phases: phase 1 focuses on the strengths and goals of the supervisee, phase 2 concentrates on patient-focused supervision, and phase 3 focuses on education, feedback, and homework.

- Solution-focused supervision begins with an exploration of the strengths and competencies of the supervisee.

- It is essential to evaluate supervisees' VIPs. These VIPs are the important elements in the system in which they work that would tell them they are being successful and doing a good job.

- Asking supervisees what they have tried that has been most helpful for their patient assists the supervisor in uncovering successes.

- Supervision is a process that is "once removed" from the patient. Asking supervisees "what your patient would say" is a linguistic technique that addresses how to maintain the focus on the patient, given that the patient is not directly involved in the supervisory process.

- Asking the supervisee to consider what the patient would say the supervisee is doing that is most helpful for him or her assists the supervisee in thinking about the patient's perspective.

- Feedback for the supervisee may include giving compliments, enumerating the positive differences discovered in the session, suggesting doing more of what works, asking what would increase the supervisee's effectiveness by one point, and encouraging trying out new questions and techniques.

- Offering education and suggestions in the form of a question maintains the nonassuming stance with the supervisee.

References

Berg IK: Family Based Services: A Solution-Focused Approach. New York, WW Norton, 1994

Briggs JR, Miller G: Success enhancing supervision. Journal of Family Psychotherapy 16:199–222, 2005

Chenven M: Community systems of care for children's mental health. Child Adolesc Psychiatr Clin N Am 19:163–174, 2010

Kilminster SM, Jolly BC: Effective supervision in clinical practice settings: a literature review. Med Educ 34:827–840, 2000

Nelson TS: Education and Training in Solution-Focused Brief Therapy. New York, Haworth, 2005

O'Hanlon WH, Weiner-Davis M: In Search of Solutions: A New Direction in Psychotherapy. New York, WW Norton, 1989

Pichot T, Dolan YM: Solution-Focused Brief Therapy: Its Effective Use in Agency Settings. Binghamton, NY Haworth, 2003

Pichot T, Smock SA: Solution-Focused Substance Abuse Treatment. New York, Routledge/Taylor & Francis Group, 2009

Sarvet BD, Wegner L: Developing effective child psychiatry collaboration with primary care: leadership and management strategies. Child Adolesc Psychiatr Clin N Am 19:139–148, 2010

Thomas FN: Solution-oriented supervision: the coaxing of expertise. The Family Journal 2:11–18, 1994

Trenhaile JD: Solution-focused supervision: returning the focus to client goals. Journal of Family Psychotherapy 16:223–228, 2005

Trepper TS, Dolan Y, McCollum EE, et al: Steve de Shazer and the future of solution-focused therapy. J Marital Fam Ther 32:133–139, 2006

Wetchler JL: Solution-focused supervision. Family Therapy 17:129–138, 1990

Winters NC, Pumariga A, Work Group on Community Child and Adolescent Psychiatry, et al: Practice parameter on child and adolescent mental health care in community systems of care. J Am Acad Child Adolesc Psychiatry 46:284–299, 2007

CHAPTER 12

Solution-Focused Consultation

Often clinicians are asked to participate as consultants in the setting of a team meeting or consultation. These consultations frequently center on diagnosis and treatment decisions, bringing pathology focus to the conversation. Solution-focused consultation utilizes the same techniques that are used in solution-focused supervision, as discussed in Chapter 11. This chapter looks more specifically at consultation involving treatment teams.

Just as with other solution-focused conversations, it is important to begin the conversation with what is working in treatment so far, so that the conversation starts off in a positive direction. This opening is followed by an exploration of the patient's VIPs (very important people) and a discussion of goals. Scaling questions are extremely useful during consultations, providing a quick assessment and incorporating multiple perspectives in a respectful and goal-oriented way while maintaining a neutral tone of agreement. Asking what makes the scale number not lower often uncovers additional strengths and resources. Asking what would raise the scale by one point helps the participants negotiate and come to agreement on the next steps needed for the client to reach his or her goals. Table 12–1 lists questions that can be asked during consultation with a team or staff.

Solution-Focused Consultation Questions

Case Illustration: Team Meeting

The following is a team meeting arranged by a young boy's therapist due to increased concerns about how Shirley (the boy's mother) was managing her

TABLE 12–1.   Solution-focused questions to ask during consultations

- What treatment and interventions have been most helpful for the patient and the family?
- What would the patient say has been most helpful for him or her so far?
- What would the family say has been most helpful for them so far?
- What have treatment providers and the family tried that has helped most for the patient and the family?
- What needs to happen to make this meeting worthwhile for the patient and the family so it is most helpful for them and not a waste of time?
- What are the best hopes for the family and treatment providers so this meeting is most helpful?
- On a scale of 1–10, where 10 is the family/patient/treatment providers are satisfied with how treatment is progressing and 1 is the opposite, where would everyone rate the progress so far?
- What makes it not lower?
- What would it take to raise it by one point?

---

mental illness and parenting demands. The psychiatrist led the team meeting. Shirley was a 35-year-old mother of four children. She was being treated for schizoaffective disorder and posttraumatic stress disorder (PTSD). She currently had living with her two younger children, a 10-year-old boy and a 2-year-old girl. Her son was treated for attention-deficit/hyperactivity disorder and PTSD, and her daughter suffered from multiple developmental delays. Her two older children had been removed several years earlier by Social Services because she had difficulties in caring for them. Shirley had recently revealed she was involved in an abusive relationship and was giving all her money and belongings to her abusive boyfriend, leaving little behind for herself or her children.

Her son's therapist initiated the team consultation because of concerns she had about Shirley's parenting ability. Included in this consultation were Shirley, her therapist, her parent partner (a lay support person for Shirley), her in-home therapist, her mental health worker, and her psychiatrist. The meeting began by having all the participants introduce themselves, including saying a little bit about their role with Shirley and how long they had been involved with the case. Shirley was then asked who her VIPs are. She identified her children and the treatment team that was present for this meeting. (Shirley had limited family support, relying primarily on her treatment team.) The following excerpt is from this team consultation.

ANNE (*psychiatrist*): Shirley, what have your treatment providers done that has been most helpful for you?
> *This question immediately focuses the consultation on what is working, rather than on diagnosis and problem exploration.*
SHIRLEY: I look forward to my appointments.

ANNE: What do you look forward to about your appointments?

SHIRLEY: They keep me busy and help me to get out of the house.

ANNE: What else has been most helpful for you in your treatment?

SHIRLEY: I don't know.

ANNE (*asking treatment providers*): What have you found that has been most helpful for Shirley in the treatment you provide?

> *This question maintains the focus on the patient while simultaneously providing opportunities to compliment her providers.*

THERAPIST: I think it helps her to have someone to bounce ideas off and give her a sense of right and wrong.

ANNE: What else do you think has been helpful for her?

THERAPIST: I think coming to my appointments helps to keep her from getting isolated. She is good about making her appointments for herself and her children.

ANNE: What have other people found has been most helpful for Shirley?

MENTAL HEALTH WORKER: I think modeling ways for her to take care of herself and then practicing this with her helps. We went out and bought make-up for her. She hadn't done something for herself in a very long time. She is a worthy person, and I want her to realize that so she can unearth what she really enjoys in her own life.

ANNE: Wow! That's great. What else has been helpful in her treatment?

IN-HOME FAMILY THERAPIST: I try to help her realize what's best for her so people won't take advantage of her. I try to help her think things through. I try to help her do practical things, like exercise her mind by reading books that she enjoys, take her kids outside and start with small changes she can make.

ANNE: I am so impressed with how many people care about you and all the hard work everyone is doing. There are already so many things that are being done that are helping Shirley and her family. I am wondering, Shirley, what are your best hopes for this meeting so you can say it was worthwhile that you came today?

> *Following the exploration of what is working in treatment, and the complimenting of the participants, the conversation is directed toward goal negotiation. The goals for the meeting are explored first by asking the patient, followed by the other participants.*

SHIRLEY: I need to learn how to budget my money.

ANNE: That can be very difficult to do. It sounds like you thought a lot about this. What have you tried to do to budget your money that has been helpful for you?

> *Asking what patients and providers have tried to do to accomplish their goals conveys the working assumption that they have already made some attempts to accomplish their goals, and perhaps had some success.*

SHIRLEY: I do pay all my bills and make sure I do that.

> *A significant strength is discovered.*

ANNE: That's fantastic. How have you been able to do that?

SHIRLEY: I have always been good at paying my bills. My problem is how many people ask me for money. I have a hard time not giving it to them. My older son calls all the time asking for my money, and my boyfriend is always harassing me for money.

Notice that she reveals an important problem she has after being complimented on her success. This often happens. When conversations are started with deposits, patients often feel more comfortable revealing their difficulties honestly and openly.

ANNE: That must be very difficult for you. How do you cope with those calls?

SHIRLEY: It is hard. Sometimes I give in, but I didn't give my boyfriend the money he asked me for today.

A positive difference is uncovered and is important to amplify.

ANNE: Was that different for you to keep the money and not give it to your boyfriend today?

SHIRLEY: Yes.

ANNE: How was that different for you?

SHIRLEY: I have given a lot of my money away to my boyfriend and my son. They harass me every day. I get scared that if I don't give my boyfriend money he will leave me, and my son always gives me all these reasons, like needing diapers and food for his young son.

ANNE: This must be very difficult for you. Was it helpful for you to keep the money and not give it to your boyfriend?

I continue to amplify this positive difference

SHIRLEY: Yes.

ANNE: How was it helpful for you?

SHIRLEY: I had money to get some clothes for my kids and didn't need to ask my brother for money. My brother told me he would stop giving me money at the end of the month.

ANNE: How have you been able to do this, not give your money away to your boyfriend?

SHIRLEY: I am sick and tired of it. I'm sick of people asking me for things and then when I need something, they don't have anything to help me.

ANNE: Of course, you have good reason to be sick of this. I am impressed how you are realizing this for yourself. I'm wondering, suppose 10 is you are confident you can budget your money and 1 is the opposite, where would you say you are now?

SHIRLEY: I'm not sure (*pause*). Maybe a 3.

ANNE: What makes it not lower for you?

SHIRLEY: I always pay all my bills.

ANNE: That's fantastic. What else makes it not lower?

SHIRLEY: My brother helps me. He reminds me to save money.

ANNE: What else makes it not lower?

SHIRLEY: I didn't give my boyfriend the money he asked for.

ANNE: That's great. You are doing a lot already. What would it take to raise it by one point?

SHIRLEY: I have to stop giving money to my older son and my boyfriend.

ANNE: What else would it take?

SHIRLEY: That they stop harassing me.

ANNE: That must be very difficult for you to manage this harassment. What have you tried that has helped?

SHIRLEY: To just not give them the money.

ANNE: How have you been able to do this?

SHIRLEY: I am tired of them.

ANNE: How would it be helpful for you to keep your money?

SHIRLEY: I would have money for furniture in my house, and clothes for my children and for emergencies.

ANNE: How else would you be able to keep your money?

SHIRLEY: I would have to say no.

ANNE: That can be very difficult. How confident are you (*addressing her treatment providers*) that Shirley can budget her money?

> *Scaling with her treatment providers brings the whole team easily and constructively into collaborative goal negotiation with the patient.*

THERAPIST: I think that she is a 6.

ANNE: What makes that not lower?

THERAPIST: She has always been good at reaching out for help and is honest. She shows up for her appointments and is always seeking advice.

ANNE: What else makes it not lower?

THERAPIST: She is insightful and notices things.

ANNE: What does Shirley notice that gives you confidence she could budget her money?

> *The same process of questioning is applied with the other participants: what makes the number not lower, what else makes it not lower, while also being mindful to incorporate the participants' exact words within questions and responses.*

The conversation continued with more scaling questions to both Shirley and the staff. The consultation concluded with compliments to both Shirley and the treatment team based on the conversation. Her therapist asked Shirley how helpful the meeting was for her on a scale of 1–10, and Shirley said 10. This confirmed to the whole team that the consultation was a success.

Solution-Focused Staff Training

Consultation can also involve staff trainings. The following case illustration exemplifies how to incorporate solution-focused consultation techniques when training and consulting to multiple staff. The same strategies are used when training multiple staff: beginning with strengths and VIPs, progressing to goal negotiation, and then asking scaling questions.

Case Illustration: Staff Training—Beginning With Staff Strengths

I was asked to do a mandatory training for all staff at a residential facility treating adolescent girls with substance abuse and co-occurring disorders, the goal being to teach staff skills in solution-focused practices. About 15 staff members were present for this training. The program was a 15-bed residential treatment facility with an average length of stay of 90 days. The age range of the patients was 13–18 years. The program was publicly funded and was suffering from financial cuts and constraints, resulting in exhausted staff working with very challenging patients for minimal pay. I began the training by appreciating all the hard work the staff do and the compassion and commitment they demonstrate when working with these patients. This phase of training is analogous to phase one of supervision as described in the previous chapter. Asking the staff what they have tried that has been most helpful for their patients followed this. Starting in this way commences with conversational deposits of tasks that the staff are already having success with, mirroring the process of beginning with conversational deposits with patients. People are people, and starting with deposits and strengths early in the conversation promotes the alliance with the staff you are working with.

ANNE: Thank you all for coming here. I know for many of you this required coming in on your day off and taking time out of your busy lives. This is very important work you all do and takes tremendous effort, dedication, passion, and commitment on your part. I hope that I can be helpful for you today so that this time will be useful for you and you can say that it was worthwhile that you came. I would like to start by asking you what skills and strategies you have found most helpful in working with your patients?

STAFF [*indicates comments from various staff members*]: I think listening.

ANNE: What else?

STAFF: Empathy.

ANNE: What do you mean empathy?

STAFF: That the patients feel heard and understood.

ANNE: Of course. What is it that you do that helps your patients feel heard and understood?

STAFF: Showing them you care.

ANNE: What do you do that shows them you care?

STAFF: Listening to them and helping them.

ANNE: What else do you do that helps them feel heard and understood?

STAFF: That we teach them skills and actually spend time doing things with them, even if it's just playing a game and taking a walk with them.

ANNE: So, doing things with them and teaching them. I am so impressed by all the skills you already have that are helping your patients. You are an amazing staff. How did you learn these skills?

STAFF: By experience and trying to see what works. By trial and error and not giving up.

This conversation continued, with the result that many skills and strengths were identified with the staff. This order of questioning is similar to that presented with patients, beginning by asking what skills and talents they have found most helpful in working with their patients. After asking what skills and strategies the staff found most helpful when working with patients, I asked what they thought their patients would say they do that was most helpful for them. This phase of training is analogous to phase 2 of patient-centered supervision. This order of questioning was intentional. First the strengths of the staff were identified, and then questions were asked that brought the patients into the conversation. Let's continue to see what happened.

> ANNE: What do you suppose your patients would say you have done that has been most helpful for them?
>
> STAFF (*pause*): I think when we're able to listen. Listening is really important.
>
> ANNE: What do you suppose would tell your patients that you are really listening to them?
>
> STAFF: When you reflect what they say so they know you are really listening.
>
> ANNE: What do you mean "reflecting"?
>
> STAFF: That you use their words so they really feel heard.
>
> ANNE: What else do you think your patients would say you have done that is most helpful for them?
>
> STAFF: Talking to them and processing with them.
>
> ANNE: What else?
>
> STAFF: Staying calm and trying to really understand them.
>
> ANNE: Staying calm can be very difficult when working with these kids. It is probably one of the most challenging skills to learn. How are you able to stay calm when working with these kids?
>
> STAFF: It's hard. We have a good team here and work hard together.
>
> ANNE: I am sure it must be hard for you. What tells you that you are a good team?
>
> STAFF: We try and really work together and listen to each other's ideas.

The conversation continued with the focus on what staff thought "their patients would say" has been most helpful for the patients. These two aspects of the consultation uncovered tremendous skills and strengths of the staff that many were as yet unaware of. Solution-focused conversations with patients begin with discovering strengths and skills, and this is the same for working with staff. After enough time was spent making deposits with the staff, I began with goal negotiation, asking what their best hopes were for the training. Let's continue with the conversation.

> ANNE: I am so impressed with all the skills and strategies you all have in working with these challenging clients. Your ability to listen, to process with the girls, to teach them many skills, all while remaining calm, is amazing. I am wondering what your best hopes are for this time together so you can say it was helpful and worthwhile for you to come here?
>
> STAFF: It can get so frustrating with these kids. They argue about everything and complain and can be so disrespectful. It's exhausting.
>
> ANNE: Of course, these are very challenging kids. This must be exhausting and frustrating for you. What would tell you that this time together was useful and helpful for you?

STAFF: I think if we learned how to handle the patients so we weren't arguing about things.

ANNE: What would you hope to do instead of arguing with them?

STAFF: Engage with them and build a treatment alliance.

ANNE: What else would be helpful for you during this time?

STAFF: To have some tools for what to do when they refuse to do things. It's so hard to deal with them when they refuse to get out of bed, refuse do their chores, or use such disrespectful language.

ANNE: Of course, this must be very difficult for you. What else would be helpful to make this time worthwhile for you?

STAFF: We have to balance the needs of the patients to want to talk with us individually while taking care of them as a group. There are only three of us on one shift, so when one person is pulled away, the other staff are cut short. I can tell that the patients seem to benefit from these times, but there just isn't the time or staff available to give them what they need.

ANNE: This must be so difficult for you to balance the needs of the individual patients, the group needs, and your co-workers' needs all while trying to keep everyone safe. What have you tried to do to cope with this?

STAFF: After working here for years and struggling with one particular patient who would hide razor blades, tell me she had secrets, then not talk about them and tell me she wasn't sure she could keep herself safe, I learned by trial and error what didn't work.

ANNE: What did you eventually learn that did work or helped a bit?

STAFF: I told her it must be tough for her, and then I would ask her what she needed to do now in this moment to get through the evening and have a better day tomorrow.

ANNE: Wow, that's a fantastic question! Every word of your question was amazing. What do the rest of you think this staff member did in this question that was helpful?

STAFF: She acknowledged that it was tough.

ANNE: What else?

STAFF: She asked her what she needed.

ANNE: What else?

STAFF: She focused on today and what she could do.

ANNE: That's a lot. I am impressed about how you developed this question. That takes a lot of skill.

Following this goal negotiation conversation, the staff was asked to participate in a compliment exercise. This exercise is a powerful activity in which a staff member is asked to complain for 2 minutes and the rest of the staff is asked to respond to these complaints only with compliments. In this particular training, the staff member acted like an angry and defiant adolescent ranting about how much she hated being there, how all the rules were stupid, how she has no desire to get clean, "F this" and "F that," how all she cares about is getting out of here and having a cigarette, and when can she call her probation officer to get her out of here. The staff initially sat dumbfounded as to how they could possibly respond to this diatribe, but once they got going, the whole whiteboard with filled with the compliments they had identified. They were able to comment on her ability to vocalize what she wanted, advocate for her needs, stay here and not run from the program in spite of her desire to leave and go and use, her goals to stay out of trouble, and her connections with her probation officer, to name a few. This exercise helped the staff see how difficult it is to identify compliments, but when they are listened for, they can be discovered.

The compliment exercise was followed by a discussion on how to build a yes-set with clients. The yes-set, as discussed in previous chapters, is established by creating as much agreement as possible between the client and the clinician. One way to help staff learn this skill is to have them practice the following emotional yes-set exercise. This exercise begins by asking the staff if there is any situation or patient that they are struggling with and would like help with. This offers them an opportunity to get consultation and support, while also providing them an opportunity to learn solution-focused techniques pertinent to their particular needs. During this particular training, one staff member brought up a very difficult situation in which one of the patients was refusing to go to a required group held outside the facility. This created significant stress for the staff as they tried to meet the needs of the patients who would benefit from attending this group while also managing the patient refusing to attend and all the staffing and safety issues surrounding this decision. After the staff member had discussed this case for 2 minutes, the other staff were asked to provide her only with emotional yes-set responses and compliments. This exercise resulted in her crying, stating how much this helped her and how she "got" how to do this. The training continued by having the staff, as a group, practice scaling questions with her. Following this group exercise, the staff was asked to break up into pairs. The groups were instructed to practice having one person complain and the other respond with compliments, emotional yes-set responses, and scaling questions. They were also instructed to practice asking each other who their VIPs are and what they most appreciate about them. Following these exercises, the staff were debriefed about what was helpful about these exercises.

In working with staff, it is important to address their specific goals, respectfully addressing their stated needs. For these staff members, it was important for them to learn how to perform brief 5-minute solution-focused check-ins with their patients so the simultaneous needs of individual patients, the group of patients as a whole, and the needs of the staff could be better attended to. Just as with patients, I began by asking the staff what they had tried that was helpful in these difficult situations. This set in motion a conversation that focused on uncovering and discovering solutions that the staff had already had success with, producing many useful strategies. One staff member commented that she would let a patient know that what he or she had to say was very important and she could spend a few minutes with him or her but also needed to take care of the group, and she would offer to check in with the patient several times during that shift.

Scaling questions were also explored as a quick way to negotiate goals with patients. For example, scaling could be applied to safety, coping ability, ability to remain calm and to get their needs met, and how well they were managing cravings. These questions could be followed by what makes the number not lower, and what else makes it not lower, and then what it would take to make it one point higher. In this way, scaling questions were offered as a tool to rapidly negotiate and come to an agreement on goals with the staff, while also helping to uncover additional strengths.

The staff also requested help with how to bring these mini-check-ins to a close. They were invited to consider how complimenting their patients, appreciating their patients' efforts to talk with them, recommending their patients do more of what's working, and paying attention to when their scaling number goes up by one point can all be useful to bring these conversations to a close briefly and productively.

It was interesting to observe that the girls noticed the staff interacting with them differently following the solution-focused staff trainings. One patient said it most eloquently: "The way I grew up, if I did something good, no one noticed, so I got used to no one noticing. Here the staff notice when I do positive things. It has motivated me, improved my mood, and helped me get through the day."

As can be seen, solution-focused conversational techniques can be used in a myriad of settings. This is because the skill involves conversation, and conversation is what people do. People are people! Whether they are old or young, male or female. By this time, you are well on your way to becoming a solution-focused clinician, being able to work with a variety of patients in many different settings, and providing supervision and training to staff. The last chapter will consider yet another setting.

Learning Exercise: Staff Compliment and Scaling Exercise

Challenge staff to spend time listening for opportunities to compliment their colleagues. If there is time, have staff pair off and practice the compliment exercise with each other. Ask the pairs to also practice the following scaling questions: Supposing 10 is you are satisfied with the work you are doing and 1 is the opposite, where would you say you are now? What makes it not lower? What else makes it not lower? What would it take to raise it by one point? How satisfied do you suppose your patients would say they are with the treatment you provide on a scale of 1–10? What was this training exercise like for you? Suggest that the staff members try to compliment both patients and staff on their next work shift and see whether doing this was helpful for them and their patients.

KEY POINTS

- Solution-focused consultations begin by asking what has been most helpful for the patient and family in their treatment so far.

- Solution-focused consultations ask the treatment providers about what they have tried that has been most helpful for their patient in treatment so far.

- It is important to ask patients and treatment providers what their best hopes are for the consultation and what would tell them the meeting is worthwhile and not a waste of time.

- Scaling questions can quickly add many perspectives in a brief time.

- Amplifying scaling questions with both patients and treatment providers details more goals and successes.

- Asking treatment providers to consider what their "patients would say" they have done that has been most helpful for treatment maintains the focus on the patient's needs.

- It is important to begin staff trainings with direct compliments and indirect questions that explore what staff have found most helpful in working with their patients.

CHAPTER 13

Conclusion

Becoming solution focused offers both a philosophy and a skill set for helping people move forward in their life. It takes discipline and hard work to notice and listen with the proverbial "third ear," ask useful questions, provide meaningful and genuine compliments, and co-create conversations so people can draw on their own strengths to help themselves. These conversations help not only the patient but also the clinician, creating hope, confidence, and optimism for all parties involved. These are privileged and extraordinary conversations.

I will end with a personal story about using solution-focused skills in my own life. We all love, and need, to complain. I am no exception.

The story begins when I was trying to complete the last phases of this book while needing to accomplish a whole list of demands on my daily to-do list. I was exhausted, irritable, and in no mood to argue with my children about the need to practice their instruments. My children have many strengths and talents, but practicing ungrudgingly is not one of them. My efforts to encourage my 11-year-old, Brandon, to practice are often fraught with nagging, arguing, and negotiating. My 13-year-old son, Ethan, frequently complains (and rightly so), "Here we go again, Brandon and mom arguing about practicing." On this particular day, my older son approached me and said: "Mom, you know, for writing a book on solution-focused therapy, you really aren't being very solution focused."

He of course was absolutely right! I have found that sometimes it can be most difficult to remain solution focused in our own personal lives, with our own children, spouses, and loved ones, especially when we are feeling worried, harried, and exhausted. His statement made me pause and reflect, and I decided on a whim to ask him whether he would be willing to help

213

me out. He agreed, always being up for "lively conversation," as he describes it. I asked him whether he would be open to trying out the compliment exercise that I had written about in the book, in which someone complains for two minutes and the other person can only respond with compliments. He was up for the challenge. I asked whether he would be willing to be the complimenter, and me, the complainer, given my level of frustration and irritability. He agreed.

I began to complain about how I wished that Brandon would practice more willingly, about how hard it is for him to focus, and how sad and frustrated this made me feel because it got in the way of him being as successful as I knew he could be. Why did I have to ask him so many times to get started? Why did he need to argue about everything I asked him to do? I grumbled about how annoyed, discouraged, and disheartened I felt, suffering through this routine on a daily basis. I went on for a full two minutes and then turned to Ethan. He looked at me dumbstruck and said, "This is going to be hard." Again, he was of course, correct, and I concurred, but encouraged him to give it a try, please, "for all of our sakes."

You know the saying, when mom isn't happy, no one is. Both my children know this only too well! He started slowly but quickly gained momentum. He embarked by saying how I don't give up on Brandon. That I keep trying no matter what, and that Brandon perseveres. He mentioned that we seem alike in this way. He went on to say how hard it must be for both of us, and that sometimes Brandon does practice without complaining. He commended Brandon on how well he plays a lot of the time and what a good lesson he had last week. He was amazed that I stayed calm for as long as I did. He appreciated my efforts not just in helping Brandon, but also with his own music. This interchange did not last long, maybe a total of five minutes.

The consequences of this brief conversation were amazing. The first thing I noticed was that both Ethan and I were smiling. This in itself was somewhat of a miracle. I felt more relaxed, more hopeful, and more confident that I could remain unflustered and cool-headed. I proceeded to compliment Ethan on how incredibly helpful this was for me and what a great job he did at finding all these compliments in such a difficult situation. He felt proud. I felt proud of him.

The story does not end here. I went back to my son Brandon and asked him whether he would give his mother another chance at trying to help him practice. By this time, we were both more composed, and he agreed. I began by complimenting him on how far he had come with the musical piece he was playing, how difficult it was, and how proud I was of him that he was able to learn so many challenging songs and work through the hard parts without giving up. I praised him for how he was able to calm down and stop himself from "flipping out" (as he describes this) when things get hard. He proceeded to practice without arguing, and worked diligently and conscientiously. We both complimented each other on our ability to remain calm. I asked him how helpful I was to him on a scale of 1–10, and he said 10. I asked him what made the number not lower, and he said "Mom, when you are calm, it helps me stay calm." We both smiled and I asked him for a hug.

We all felt better. Ethan felt better about his skill at complimenting, helping out, voicing his needs and frustration about practicing, and having his needs responded to. Brandon felt proud of his ability to remain calm, work through conflict with his mother, stay focused without "flipping out," and progress with his musical piece. I felt proud of both my children and all the skills they were learning. We together had figured out a different solution to what was a chronic and daily problem. I went on to tell my husband all about it. He smiled, being all too familiar with this situation. He asked me what worked, and what I needed to do more of. I talked about my need to stay calm, compliment my children, and manage my own frustration. He asked me how confident I was on a scale of 1–10 that I could keep this up. I said maybe a 6 or 7, but definitely up from a 2.

I remember what Steve de Shazer said: if it works, do more of it, and if it doesn't, do something different. This is the core of the solution-focused model. This may sound simple, but simple does not mean easy—something of which I often remind my children, my patients, and myself.

Solution-focused therapy is a conversational discipline that can be learned and used in myriad settings. This is because conversation involves talking with people, and people are people. My hope is that this book has been useful for you, and that you will try a few of these techniques for staying solution focused with the patients and the people in your life, deciding for yourself whether it works.

APPENDIX

Rating Scales

Mood Assessment

Scaled item	Scale of 1–10
Rate your happiness from 1–10, where 10 is you are happy all the time and 1 is the opposite.	1—2—3—4—5—6—7—8—9—10
Rate your confidence that things will work out for you, where 10 is you are confident they will work out all the time and 1 is the opposite.	1—2—3—4—5—6—7—8—9—10
Rate how well you do things right, where 10 is you always do things right and 1 is the opposite.	1—2—3—4—5—6—7—8—9—10
Rate how much fun you have doing things, where 10 is you have a lot of fun doing many things and 1 is the opposite.	1—2—3—4—5—6—7—8—9—10
Rate how often you do the right thing, where 10 is you do the right thing all the time and 1 is the opposite.	1—2—3—4—5—6—7—8—9—10
Rate how confident you are that good things will happen to you, where 10 is you are sure that good things will happen to you and 1 is the opposite.	1—2—3—4—5—6—7—8—9—10
Rate how much you like yourself, where 10 is you like yourself a lot and 1 is the opposite.	1—2—3—4—5—6—7—8—9—10
Rate how much you think that good things are a result of your behavior, where 10 is you believe many good things are a result of your behavior and 1 is the opposite.	1—2—3—4—5—6—7—8—9—10
Rate how strong your reasons for living are, where 10 is you have many reasons to live and 1 is the opposite.	1—2—3—4—5—6—7—8—9—10
Rate how often you feel happy and do not feel like crying, where 10 is you feel happy all the time and 1 is the opposite.	1—2—3—4—5—6—7—8—9—10

Scaled item	Scale of 1–10
Rate how well you are able to let things go, where 10 is you are able to let things go and 1 is the opposite.	1—2—3—4—5—6—7—8—9—10
Rate how much you like being with people, where 10 is you enjoy being with people all the time and 1 is the opposite.	1—2—3—4—5—6—7—8—9—10
Rate how easily you can make up your mind and make decisions, where 10 is it is easy to make up your mind and make decisions and 1 is the opposite.	1—2—3—4—5—6—7—8—9—10
Rate how good you feel about your looks, where 10 is you like the way you look and 1 is the opposite.	1—2—3—4—5—6—7—8—9—10
Rate how easy it is to get your schoolwork done, where 10 is it is easy to get yourself to do your schoolwork and 1 is the opposite.	1—2—3—4—5—6—7—8—9—10
Rate how well you sleep at night, where 10 is you sleep very well at night and 1 is the opposite.	1—2—3—4—5—6—7—8—9—10
Rate how much energy you have during the day, where 10 is you have all the energy you need during the day and 1 is the opposite.	1—2—3—4—5—6—7—8—9—10
Rate how well you eat, where 10 is you feel like eating most days and 1 is the opposite.	1—2—3—4—5—6—7—8—9—10
Rate how comfortable you feel in terms of feeling pain free, where 10 is you do not experience aches and pains and 1 is the opposite.	1—2—3—4—5—6—7—8—9—10
Rate how well you feel connected to others, where 10 is you feel well connected to others and 1 is the opposite.	1—2—3—4—5—6—7—8—9—10

Scaled item	Scale of 1–10
Rate how often you have fun at school, where 10 is you have fun all the time at school and 1 is the opposite.	1—2—3—4—5—6—7—8—9—10
Rate how good you feel about the number of friends you have, where 10 is you feel you have plenty of good friends and 1 is the opposite.	1—2—3—4—5—6—7—8—9—10
Rate how good you feel about your schoolwork, where 10 is you feel very good about your schoolwork and 1 is the opposite.	1—2—3—4—5—6—7—8—9—10
Rate how you feel about yourself compared to other kids, where 10 is you feel very good about yourself and 1 is the opposite.	1—2—3—4—5—6—7—8—9—10
Rate how confident you are that somebody loves you, where 10 is you are very confident that somebody loves you and 1 is the opposite.	1—2—3—4—5—6—7—8—9—10
Rate how cooperative you are when asked to do things, where 10 is you are very cooperative and 1 is the opposite.	1—2—3—4—5—6—7—8—9—10
Rate how good you are at getting along with others and remaining calm in times of conflict, where 10 is you are very good at getting along with others and remaining calm in times of conflict and 1 is the opposite.	1—2—3—4—5—6—7—8—9—10

Child Attention Profile

Scaled item	Scale of 1–10
Rate how you well you are able to follow through on tasks, where 10 is you are able to follow through on all tasks and 1 is the opposite.	1—2—3—4—5—6—7—8—9—10
Rate how well you are able to maintain attention to task, where 10 is you are able to maintain your attention for a long period and 1 is the opposite.	1—2—3—4—5—6—7—8—9—10
Rate how good you are at keeping your body calm and being able to sit still, where 10 is you are able to sit still and keep your body calm all the time and 1 is the opposite.	1—2—3—4—5—6—7—8—9—10
Rate how well you are able to keep your body calm, where 10 is you able to keep calm all the time and 1 is the opposite.	1—2—3—4—5—6—7—8—9—10
Rate how good you are at maintaining your focus on what is happening in the moment, where 10 is you can maintain your focus and 1 is the opposite.	1—2—3—4—5—6—7—8—9—10
Rate how good you are at thinking before acting and maintaining your self-control, where 10 is you are good at thinking before acting and maintaining your control all the time and 1 is the opposite.	1—2—3—4—5—6—7—8—9—10
Rate how well you are able to follow directions, where 10 is you are good at following directions all the time and 1 is the opposite.	1—2—3—4—5—6—7—8—9—10
Rate how good you are at waiting your turn and waiting to be called on by the teacher, where 10 is you are good at waiting to speak up until asked and when it is your turn and 1 is the opposite.	1—2—3—4—5—6—7—8—9—10
Rate how neat you are with your work, where 10 is your work is very neat all the time and 1 is the opposite.	1—2—3—4—5—6—7—8—9—10

Index

Page numbers printed in *boldface* type refer to tables or figures.